Inside Public
Psychiatry

Inside Public Psychiatry

Selby C. Jacobs, MD, MPH

2011
PEOPLE'S MEDICAL PUBLISHING HOUSE–USA
SHELTON, CONNECTICUT

People's Medical Publishing House-USA
2 Enterprise Drive, Suite 509
Shelton, CT 06484
Tel: 203-402-0646
Fax: 203-402-0854
E-mail: info@pmph-usa.com

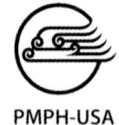

PMPH-USA

11 12 13 14/PMPH/9 8 7 6 5 4 3 2 1

ISBN-13: 978-1-60795-113-1
ISBN-10: 1-60795-113-4

Printed in China by People's Medical Publishing House
Editor: Linda H. Mehta; Copyeditor/Typesetter: Newgen; Cover designers: Bruno Bissonnette and Mary McKeon

Library of Congress Cataloging-in-Publication Data

Jacobs, Selby, 1939-
 Inside public psychiatry / Selby Jacobs.
   p. ; cm.
 Includes bibliographical references and index.
 ISBN-13: 978-1-60795-113-1 (alk. paper)
 ISBN-10: 1-60795-113-4 (alk. paper)

1. Connecticut Mental Health Center. 2. Community mental health services—Connecticut. 3. Academic medical centers—Connecticut. 4. Community psychiatry—Connecticut—History. I. Title.

 [DNLM: 1. Connecticut Mental Health Center. 2. Community Mental Health Services—history—Connecticut. 3. Academic Medical Centers—history—Connecticut. 4. Community Psychiatry—history—Connecticut. 5. History, 20th Century—Connecticut. 6. History, 21st Century—Connecticut. WM 11 AC8]
 RA790.65.C8J33 2011
 362.2'209746—dc22

                                           2010052005

Sales and Distribution

Canada
McGraw-Hill Ryerson Education
Customer Care
300 Water St
Whitby, Ontario L1N 9B6
Canada
Tel: 1-800-565-5758
Fax: 1-800-463-5885
www.mcgrawhill.ca

Foreign Rights
People's Medical Publishing House
Suzanne Robidoux, Copyright Sales
Manager
International Trade Department
No. 19, Pan Jia Yuan Nan Li
Chaoyang District
Beijing 100021
P.R. China
Tel: 8610-59787337
Fax: 8610-59787336
www.pmph.com/en/

Japan
United Publishers Services Limited
1-32-5 Higashi-Shinagawa
Shinagawa-ku, Tokyo 140-0002
Japan
Tel: 03-5479-7251
Fax: 03-5479-7307
Email: kakimoto@ups.co.jp

United Kingdom, Europe, Middle East, Africa
McGraw Hill Education
Shoppenhangers Road
Maidenhead
Berkshire, SL6 2QL
England
Tel: 44-0-1628-502500
Fax: 44-0-1628-635895
www.mcgraw-hill.co.uk

Singapore, Thailand, Philippines, Indonesia,
Vietnam, Pacific Rim, Korea
McGraw-Hill Education
60 Tuas Basin Link
Singapore 638775
Tel: 65-6863-1580
Fax: 65-6862-3354
www.mcgraw-hill.com.sg

Australia, New Zealand, Papua New Guinea, Fiji, Tonga, Solomon Islands, Cook Islands
Woodslane Pty Limited
Unit 7/5 Vuko Place
Warriewood NSW 2102
Australia
Tel: 61-2-9970-5111
Fax: 61-2-9970-5002
www.woodslane.com.au

Brazil
SuperPedido Tecmedd
Beatriz Alves, Foreign Trade
Department
R. Sansao Alves dos Santos, 102 | 7th
floor
Brooklin Novo
Sao Paolo 04571-090
Brazil
Tel: 55-16-3512-5539
www.superpedidotecmedd.com.br

India, Bangladesh, Pakistan, Sri Lanka, Malaysia
CBS Publishers
4819/X1 Prahlad Street 24
Ansari Road, Darya Ganj, New Delhi-110002
India
Tel: 91-11-23266861/67
Fax: 91-11-23266818
Email:cbspubs@vsnl.com

People's Republic of China
People's Medical Publishing House
International Trade Department
No. 19, Pan Jia Yuan Nan Li
Chaoyang District
Beijing 100021
P.R. China
Tel: 8610-67653342
Fax: 8610-67691034
www.pmph.com/en/

This book is dedicated to the people served by the Connecticut Mental Health Center and to the clinicians, educators, and investigators who serve them.

Table of Contents

Foreword

Like most people who have trained at the Connecticut Mental Health Center (CMHC), it holds a special place in my heart. An urban community mental health center that was created at the height of the Great Society programs, it is run by the Yale Department of Psychiatry for the State of Connecticut's Department of Mental Health and Addiction Services. It is a principal training site for the Yale Department of Psychiatry. It is also the jewel in the clinical crown for both parent organizations and has benefited over its lifetime as an institution from the leaders appointed to head it.

Since opening in 1966, the CMHC has served the public by caring for people with mental illness, evaluating the nature of mental illnesses and treatments for them, and teaching about it. By telling the story of clinical services at the CMHC, *Inside Public Psychiatry* complements a previous volume published on the fortieth anniversary of the institution (Jacobs, Griffith, 2007). Given the central role of the CMHC in the Yale Department of Psychiatry and its commitment to clinical care, research, and education, it is no accident that this is the second work in recent years in which CMHC figures prominently. The first book, *40 Years of Academic Public Psychiatry*, is a detailed history of the events and accomplishments of the academic programs in public psychiatry at the CMHC. Not only can it be read as a companion to the current work, but also one can discern in its introduction the point of departure for the present work. Reciprocally, *Inside Public Psychiatry* fleshes out an understanding of the clinical foundations of the CMHC, converting the somewhat hollow shell in the account of academic programs into a whole picture. In this way, this present volume extends the personal, and at times idiosyncratic, academic history of CMHC as described in *40 Years*, and uses that history to serve as an ongoing "case history" for the larger trends in public psychiatry.

The author of *Inside Public Psychiatry*, Dr. Selby Jacobs, was the head of the CMHC from 1996 to 2009. He has spent much of his professional career in public psychiatry, and his decades-long service affords him the "long view" so indispensable in a book with such ambitions as this one. For his ambition is grand, in making sense of the developments in public psychiatry in the past five decades and in his use of the history of CMHC as an illustrative guide.

Serendipity has clearly favored the writing of *Inside Public Psychiatry*. There is no doubt that we find ourselves in a very exciting time for public psychiatry. However, the future is uncertain and the implications for organizations like the CMHC, in the context of mental health parity and health care reform, are also obscure. It is in this context that the author's use of the parallel narratives of the nation in general and the CMHC in particular can serve the reader well. Interested readers in the field of public psychiatry can perform a similar, and very illuminating, exercise for their own institutions, for both the past and the future.

I would like to end with a few more words about Dr. Jacobs. He was, and still is, an extraordinary steward of the mission of public psychiatry—at the CMHC, at Yale, and in national organizations such as the American Psychiatric Association through its Council on Health Care Systems and Finance. He has maintained his passion for serving those citizens most in need of help, even when the gaze of psychiatry and society may have shifted to other, more seductive areas of research and advocacy. *Inside Public Psychiatry*, when it addresses the very recent changes in mental health care and funding and the directions these changes presage for the future of our profession, is a testament to the farsightedness of a collective vision that he guided for years at the CMHC.

Michael J. Sernyak, MD
Director, Connecticut Mental Health Center
Professor of Psychiatry, Yale School of Medicine
New Haven, Connecticut

Preface

After enactment of the Community Mental Health Centers Act of 1963 and the construction act that followed in 1965, the next few years saw the emergence across the country of several academic community mental health centers. Each amalgamated services, education, and research into powerful programs for the practice of public health psychiatry in the community. Now, few academic centers remain, and the Connecticut Mental Health Center (CMHC) in New Haven, Connecticut, is a prime example. This book sets out to tell the story of the CMHC over the modern era of public psychiatry.

The CMHC opened its doors in 1966 in the midst of the earliest wave of de-institutionalization. This mental health center has operated to the present through multiple periods of public psychiatry that embraced different policies in response to the needs and problems of people with chronic illness who were leaving state psychiatric hospitals and establishing lives in the community. At present the CMHC is entering a future of healthcare reform, which poses continuing challenges for sustaining, improving, and expanding services for people who are already in the system as well as those who will gain access to care. The CMHC will need to adapt in order to survive as an institution and continue to play a leading role in serving its target population. The basic premise of this book is that a historical overview of the modern era of public psychiatry at the CMHC offers a framework for understanding not only what has transpired in public psychiatry over the past half-century but also a glimpse of what the future may hold.

For many reasons introduced in Chapter 1 and traced throughout the text, the recent, approximately half-century of public psychiatry has been crucially significant for the care of people with serious mental illness and addictions in the community. Also, significant educational and scientific progress has been achieved. It is important to build on this progress and not slip back. Much is at stake as the future of care for people with serious and persistent mental illnesses and addictions and of community mental health centers is far from secure. In addition, scientific inquiry into and education about problems germane to public mental health must progress to improve the range and quality of care for the people served in the public arena.

The rationale for writing this book was to create sequence, continuity, and context for the life and story of the CMHC and the services it offers to people suffering from mental illness and addictions. This method of historical reconstruction enabled insight into the evolution of services and practice at a particular institution in response to professional, scientific, economic, and political forces. There were background questions in mind not only about the field of public psychiatry but also about the unique institution of the CMHC. What was the story behind almost a half-century of evolution in public psychiatry? How did public psychiatry arrive at the present array of services it offers to people with serous mental illness and addictions? What was the structure and functionality of the academic CMHC that enabled it to adapt successfully, and sometimes abysmally, as the social and economic environment of care changed. How well did public psychiatry care for people with serious illnesses? How would public psychiatry adapt to meet the needs of its target population in the revolutionary times that lie ahead as a result of the historical achievement of nondiscriminatory psychiatric insurance coverage and the tidal wave of previously uninsured people seeking access to mental health care under health care reform? While developing this story, a few principles were paramount. One was to keep the care of people with serious mental illness in focus as the fundamental outcome of public psychiatry. Another was to highlight the potent and essential contributions of academic institutions in public psychiatry, which combine services, education, and research and consider the future of these institutions through the concrete example of the CMHC. This account was conceived as a starting point in a process in which others would add their facts, perspectives, analysis, and interpretations to the history, thereby enriching and validating the story.

This parochial account of public psychiatry at the CMHC is a particular instance that has universal implications for those invested in institutions devoted to academic public health psychiatry. Even this assertion is overly restrictive, as this specific case example also illuminates non-academic community mental health centers. Further, the narrative holds interest for both the governmental sector of state-owned and -operated institutions, such as the CMHC, and the private nonprofit sector, which is larger by far. In addition, the historical perspective on the CMHC and public psychiatry developed in this book serves as a useful context, beyond management of budgets, human resources, quality assurance, and expertise in clinical, educational, and research operations, for leading and managing institutions for public psychiatry. It offers depth and context for decisions that guide the life of an institution. Hopefully, this text creates a useful framework for considering the future now being shaped by parity of health insurance benefits for people with mental illness and addictions and the expanded access to mental health care under health care reform. In short, the concrete example of the CMHC, its story, and insights into the field of public psychiatry has wide applications.

This historical overview, with a focus on evolving policies, the consequences for services on the ground, and the care of people with serious mental illness across the entire period of modern public psychiatry, differs from previous books. Other texts, which are cited in subsequent chapters, include books on community psychiatry, which was the first phase of the modern era, books on the history of mental health policy, articles on the history and specific aspects of public psychiatry, and selected examples of key legislation during the modern era. None have traced the history of a particular institution as it evolved services for people with serious mental illness and addictions in response to professional, scientific, economic, and political forces. None yet have considered the choices facing public psychiatry as it projects into the future.

This story of public psychiatry and the CMHC will be of interest to psychiatrists working in the public sector. These psychiatrists make up about one-third of the 40,000 membership of the American Psychiatric Association. More than another quarter of psychiatrists, who work part-time in the public sector, are puzzled by how it operates. In the broadest sense, this book informs practice and policy formation for public psychiatry. The system view offered in the book informs clinical practice. Further, the book will serve as a useful text in educational programs for advanced medical and graduate students of public psychiatry. By illustrating the operations of an institution for public psychiatry, the book may be of interest to people with mental illness, their families, and others concerned with services for themselves. Also, mental health workers from European and Asian countries might apply the lessons of this American example to the problems they face in their own countries.

This contribution to the literature on modern public psychiatry builds on a foundation that is essential for understanding practice and progress and intends to add to understanding of this essential domain of psychiatric practice, education and inquiry.

—Selby Jacobs, MD, MPH

Acknowledgments

Many thanks to Mr. Robert Cole, Dr. Wayne Dailey, Ms. Martha Mitchell, and Dr. Michael Sernyak for reading an earlier version of this book and offering useful substantive and editorial comments. Also, thank you to Dr. Stephanie Farber for editorial suggestions about the conceptual design and style of the text. Finally, thanks to Ms. Linda Mehta, MALS of PMPH-USA and to Ms. Molly Morrison and her staff of Newgen Imaging and Data Services for final editing in preparation for publication.

The Significance of Public Psychiatry and an Overview

"Let me recite what history teaches. History teaches."
—Gertrude Stein, in *If I Told Him*, 1923

Over the almost 50 years of modern public psychiatry, what were the immediate and longer range public responses to the waves of patients now living in community rather than state hospitals? How did these public responses change over the modern era since the paradigm-shifting Community Mental Health Act of 1963 (CMHA)? What were the new institutions, called community mental health centers, that rose up to offer community-based services? What role, if any, did academic programs play in the evolution of services? How did people with acute and chronic psychiatric illnesses enter and traverse the system of community-based services at different stages of evolution? What services were available for them? What does the history of the modern period of public psychiatry portend for the future of public services?

This book traces the development of the Connecticut Mental Health Center (CMHC), an academic community mental health center in New Haven, Connecticut, through the modern era of public psychiatry. Conversely, the book offers a perspective on modern mental health policy as viewed through the lens of this particular community mental health center. The CMHC, an academic, state owned and operated institution that opened in 1966, faced the challenges and policy issues of each period in the modern era. In response to deinstitutionalization, each period at the CMHC contributed essential elements to community services in New Haven. In tracking these developments, especially as they relate to people with serious mental illness, the text offers brief case examples from the CMHC. The narrative concludes with a view of future directions for services and public psychiatry at the CMHC and, by extension, for the whole field. The discussion of mental health policies and the accruing, community-based services and systems lends universal interest and appeal to an otherwise parochial story of one academic institution.

MODERN PUBLIC PSYCHIATRY AND DEINSTITUTIONALIZATION

The underlying theme for the modern era of public psychiatry is the deinstitutionalization of psychiatric patients from state hospitals. Many of the discharged patients had lived there for years, were chronically ill, and had few independent skills for living in the community. Starting in 1956, during the next 40 years, over 450,00 patients were discharged from state psychiatric hospitals in the United States, many of which were subsequently closed (see Figure 1-1).

Upon discharge, the social and professional challenge became one of caring for these patients in the community.

The professional, political, and economic forces behind deinstitutionalization were manifold. Central to them was a new, optimistic, post–World War II clinical ideology of treating people with acute mental illnesses in the community. Experience in treating soldiers in combat at the front lines bred these beliefs. Echoes of the mental hygiene movement in the early twentieth century were present. Early evaluation, treatment, and prevention through crisis intervention were part of the new perspective.

In addition to the new ideology, the cost of state psychiatric hospitals was a burden for the states. The quality of care was poor, leading to the federal National Mental Illness and Health Act of 1955. In 1961 a national commission formed by this act published its recommendations in a report entitled "Action for Mental Health." This report coincided roughly with the election of President John F. Kennedy. The Kennedy administra-

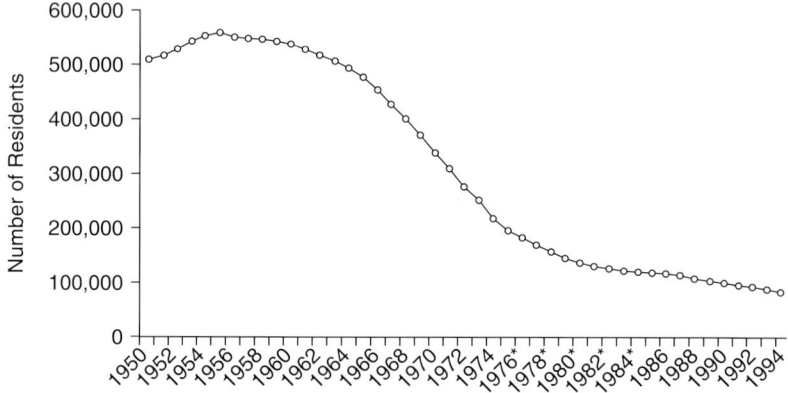

Figure 1-1 Resident patients in U.S. state and county mental hospitals at the end of each year, 1950 to 1994 (Mandershied et al., 2000).

tion adopted the new perspective and recommendations for reform, and in 1963 Congress enacted the Community Mental Health Act.

The discovery of antipsychotic drugs, beginning in 1955, also gave impetus to the new movement. Antidepressant drugs followed soon after. Lithium for manic-depressive illness entered practice in 1969. Pharmacologic treatments gave psychiatrists new tools for the treatment of mental illness in the community. Though it would take many years to put in place the full array of community services necessary for care in the community, great optimism prevailed at the opening of the modern era.

Not least among the variables enabling the modern era of public psychiatry was the enactment of Medicare and Medicaid in 1965. These health and social welfare benefits made it possible for people to live in the community with chronically illness, which often impaired their ability to work.

FOUR PERIODS OF MODERN PUBLIC PSYCHIATRY

To understand the modern era of public psychiatry, it is helpful to delineate four somewhat overlapping periods. They are:

(1) the community mental health movement from 1963-82;
(2) the development of community-based services and systems for individuals with serious mental illness from 1982-93;
(3) the mainstreaming of mental health and social welfare benefits, especially under Medicaid for people with serious mental illness, from 1993-2003, and
(4) the current period of transformation, since 2003.

The current period, which encompasses the integration of mental health and primary care, can be seen as an outgrowth of mainstreaming. The current period of transformation may be transitioning into a new period of public psychiatry under health care reform.

Alternate issues—such as translation of scientific discovery into practice, recovery from illness, and the rise of Medicaid—qualify as major themes that might be considered alternatives to the choices for organizing the modern era. Each of the four periods is characterized by pursuit of certain policy goals, sometimes in reaction to the previous period, as in the case of system development; sometimes as an extension of a previous period, such as transformation, and sometimes as an outgrowth of political and social challenges, as in mainstreaming. This book examines the specific problems faced by each of these periods and the mental health policies that were developed to deal with them. During each period, innovative community-based services emerged to finally arrive at a contemporary, broad array of services for people with mental illnesses and addictions.

THE SIGNIFICANCE OF PUBLIC PSYCHIATRY

The significance of public psychiatry is best understood one person at a time. For example, a man, who has been living under a bridge in the midst of winter is brought into a shelter, eventually finds a place to live, and starts treatment to calm his chronic paranoid suspicions of others. A woman, supported by special cognitive techniques to help her cope with persistent voices in her head saying she looks bad, is able to find and hold a part-time job, receive a small paycheck, and enter community life as an employed person. A skilled therapist finally engages a man, who had periodically assaulted urgent care clinicians and had required repeated emergency procedures to restrain him. They settle into a stable, caring relationship, opening a crack in the wall of ostracism put up by everyone who had encountered him.

> The significance of public psychiatry is best understood one person at a time.

Not all interventions are success stories, however. A woman, who fears the devil in the form of her landlord, uses opiates to calm her fearful delusions, and has her two children taken away by child welfare. The children are lost in foster care and bereft. A talented woman, who is a dropout from studying drama in graduate school, begs on the city green by reciting Shakespeare. Repeatedly, she refuses to come off the streets into residential care. A charming man when well, a gifted baseball player, relapses into psychosis again, becomes threatening, and brandishes a knife in front of support staff in his apartment. He is shot to death in a confrontation with police called by frightened house managers. The stories go on. Many are not dramatic. Multiple small, daily gestures of help and friendship for people who are suffering from serious mental illness acknowledge the shared humanity of providers and recipients of care. All these experiences impel those who work in the public domain of psychiatry to go on, keep at it, try to improve and to reach as many people as possible within the resources available to them.

On a more abstract level, the significance of public psychiatry is a function of its mission as the ultimate safety net for some of society's most vulnerable individuals, those who suffer from psychiatric disorders and disabilities and cannot afford care. Thus, public psychiatry, a subspecialty of psychiatry, is a cornerstone of psychiatric, professional, and social responsibility for others. Public psychiatry fulfills a special purpose that has been recognized since the days of Dorothea Dix in the nineteenth century. Her crusade to create hospitals for the public stemmed from the moral psychiatry movement that had begin in seventeenth-century France and England.

Public psychiatry is important because American society, though periodically embarking on initiatives such as public hospital construction in the nineteenth century or the community mental health movement of the 1960s, has never sustained a commitment over time to its most disadvantaged, seriously ill members, who suffer from psychiatric disorders and disabilities. This long history of on-again off-again commitment argues for the maintaining of special attention to the needs of this segment of the population.

The size of the public psychiatry endeavor offers another perspective on its significance. Using cost data from 2001 (including Medicaid costs, and combining costs by Medicaid and by state governments) shows that 52% of all mental health and substance-abuse expenditures were in the public arena. This estimate is low, as it neither includes Medicare expenditures on individuals who qualify for Social Security Disability Insurance as a result of adjudicated disabilities, nor federal expenditures through block grants to states for community mental health (Mark et al., 2007). According to data from the Surgeon General's 1999 report on mental health, 2% of the American population received care that year in the public sector, out of 15% in the population receiving mental health care the same year (U.S. Department of Health and Human services, 1999a).

Despite its significance, the future of public psychiatry is not clear. Public psychiatrists are a minority in American psychiatry by comparison to private practitioners, academic psychiatrists, and other professional groups. While the logic of maintaining public services is strong, especially for individuals with serious mental illness, multiple forces challenge public practice, including new public and private health insurance policies, limited resources as states contend with the economic recession of 2008, competing agendas for public services, and new practices. In the circumstances of an uncertain future, it is useful to pause, consider the recent past, place public practice in the context of social, economic, and professional forces that have shaped it, and consider a vision for future development. This book sets out to fulfill that purpose.

THE CONNECTICUT MENTAL HEALTH CENTER

The CMHC is a state owned and operated, academic community mental health center located in a midsize New England urban center. A professional services contract between the State of Connecticut and Yale

University (known by the university as the faculty contract) provides for the leadership, psychiatrists, and psychologists, as well as a few other administrative positions of the CMHC. Most nurses, social workers, and plant operations staff are state employees. The three missions of the CMHC are: services, education, and science. The clinical serves are the safety net in New Haven for low-income people afflicted with acute and chronic mental illnesses and addictions. Clinical services are platforms for the education of psychiatric residents, psychology interns, and post-doctoral students from the Yale Department of Psychiatry. Nurses and social workers from surrounding schools also rotate on these services. The services are also a platform for clinical and preclinical research, based on referral into protocols and funded by grants obtained by individuals and groups of investigators.

New Haven is a city that has known the vicissitudes of urban decay and economic renewal, violent streets, public outrage and public harmony, local politics that periodically alternate between being friendly and being hostile to the CMCH, fluctuating town versus gown relations, and the persistent blight of homelessness for three decades. In the past 10 years, New Haven has been on a trajectory of revitalization, fostered in part by cooperation between the city and the university.

The CMHC occupies a building at 34 Park Street (Figure 1-2). It is on the northwest corner of the Yale medical campus, across the street

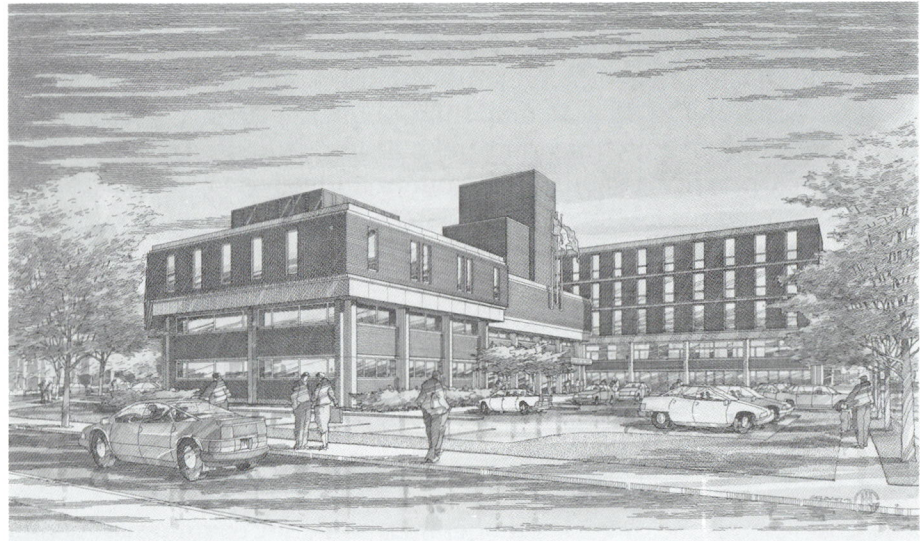

Figure 1-2 An architectural drawing of the Connecticut Mental Health Center (viewed from the southeast).

from the Smilow Cancer Center of Yale-New Haven Hospital. It is adjacent to the Hill neighborhood of New Haven, an inner city area with a diverse population. Bruce Arneill, a Yale School of Architecture graduate completed the original design for the building. Opening in 1966, the building is a 1960s-style concrete structure with a red brick façade. The main wing is a three-story, horizontal block, oriented north and south and slightly cantilevered on square concrete columns. Inside the main entrance is an urgent care service. On the second floor is a warren of ambulatory care offices, most with windows set high in the outside walls in order to protect privacy but also obstructing views of the outside. The third floor is devoted to preclinical lab space called the Ribicoff Research Facility. Forming a T on the north end of the main building is a five-story, east-west wing that houses administration, more outpatient offices on the second floor, and three hospital units on the top floors. The third floor is a clinical neuroscience research unit; the fourth is an acute unit; and the fifth is a subacute unit. In 1993, a three-story pod, the Substance Abuse Center, was opened on the south end of the main wing. In 2009, a three-story rectangular box, projecting west off the five-story building, opened to house Latino services and research labs on the top floors. The last addition created a small inner courtyard that hospitalized patients can visit. The State of Connecticut financed the original building. The state and Yale University jointly financed the two additions. The openings in 1966, 1993, and 2009 became occasions to celebrate and, with the additions, renew the partnership between the state and the university.

THE DEFINITION OF PUBLIC PSYCHIATRY

Psychiatry has paid attention to social variables and community practice for decades. Psychiatrists have known this part of their field by different names over the years. Historically, the three main denotations are social psychiatry, community psychiatry, and presently public psychiatry. Before the community mental health movement started in 1963, social psychiatry was the term that characterized that part of theory and practice that concerned itself with social variables and public health perspectives. Social psychiatrists were interested in social class and urban density as variables that might cause mental illness. They were interested in family and group interventions in order to address the social milieu of patients. They were also committed to interdisciplinary, clinical team practice. Their academic disciplines were epidemiology and clinical research, sometimes rooted in psychoanalytic theory, which prevailed at the time. The community mental health movement introduced the term community psychiatry to replace the old, social psychiatry. Community mental health professionals built on the elements of social psychiatry and embraced the policies and practices of the community mental health movement. Typically, they practiced in community mental health centers and brought services research into the academic portfolio of clinical research and epidemiology. Community mental health, and its terminology, waned after the repeal of the Mental Health Systems Act in 1981. During the period of community services and systems development, starting in 1982, the term public psychiatry rose in usage, in part as a function of the reinvigorated role of state departments of mental health. It was also a time when health insurance for psychiatric disorders was growing. Public psychiatry is part of a dichotomy. Private psychiatry, sometimes referred to as private practice, is the other part. The main distinction between these two parts is the means of financing mental health services. Commercial, third-party insurance or out of pocket payment are the means for private psychiatry. Federal or state entitlements and state general funds are the means for public psychiatry. The definition below builds on this distinction.

Even with this brief background in mind, the task of reaching a contemporary definition of public psychiatry seems daunting at first. As the public mission has evolved, the definition of public psychiatry has expanded and varied over the modern era. The professional literature on public psychiatry offers some help in establishing a contemporary definition. As a starting point, a task force of the American Association of Community Psychiatrists (AACP) published a consensus definition of community psychiatry, which was the term still in usage by the authors at the time (Brown et al., 1993). The AACP concluded that community psychiatry "is a branch of psychiatry, which emphasizes the integration of social and environmental factors with the biological and psychological components of mental health and mental illness. Community psychiatry is also a significant component of the more inclusive field of community medicine, which focuses broadly on the prevention and treatment of illness for all individuals in a given community." The community psychiatrist, who can practice independently or in an organized setting and in an interdisciplinary and collaborative manner, works as a clinician, consultant to other individuals and organizations, administrator responsible for a system, and a services researcher. Not every psychiatrist covers all these bases. Notable in this definition is the reference to community medicine, for grasping the relationship of public psychiatry to medicine and the need to consider medical models of care.

The public psychiatry group at Columbia University provided another definition, based not only on the experience of their education program but also on a survey of public psychiatrists who belonged to the AACP (Ranz, 2004). The Columbia group defined public psychiatry as "the use of clinical techniques, management skills, and evaluation strategies within established institutions serving populations with social as well as psychiatric needs: patients with severe mental illness and other major social psychiatric problems such as substance abuse, homelessness, and AIDS, as well as members of poor urban and suburban minorities."

Building on these definitions, for the purposes of the present text, the following definition of public psychiatry is used. The italics signal key elements in the definition that feature in a boiled down abstraction in the next paragraph. Public psychiatry is that part of the practice of psychiatry that is *financed* both by general funds through states' departments of mental health and reimbursement income from entitlements such as Medicaid. For disabled, chronically ill individuals, Medicare funds services, with eligibility determined by the Social Security Administration. Public psychiatry provides a safety net of services for low income mentally ill and addicted people in the community. The *practice* of public psychiatry incorporates treatment, psychosocial rehabilitation for the disabled, patient-centered recovery plans of care, integration with primary care, community supports such as housing and money management, and attention to social issues such as legal status or homelessness. Public psychiatry is practiced *in many settings*. These include mental health and addiction agencies, community behavioral health centers, residential and nursing care facilities, psychosocial rehabilitation agencies, primary care centers, and organizations offering forensic or public health programs. Practice typically occurs through *multi-disciplinary* teams. Given the multiplicity of settings and tasks, *systems knowledge*, *management skills*, and a *population perspective* are important for clinical success. Finally, public psychiatry is part of *community medicine and public health*. Public psychiatry uses not only a clinical but also a population perspective. It attends to *public health* data, epidemiologic studies, and mental health services research for the purpose of planning, evaluating, executing, and managing services.

In the above definition, the italicized key words and phrases are the essential elements in a definition of contemporary public psychiatry. This definition of public psychiatry incorporates elements from major historical and policy developments since 1963. The definition offered here is professional, medical, clinical, and administrative. It incorporates a broad, clinical and public health perspective on psychiatric disorders and clinical services. It avoids the trap of defining public psy-

> The definition offered here is professional, medical, clinical, and administrative.

chiatry in terms of the place or system where it is practiced, as these are multiple and increasingly blurred by both private and public missions. Subsequent chapters develop the perspectives opened in this definition. This brief discussion of public psychiatry is intended as a starting point for the purpose of an account of the life of the CMHC over the modern era. The reader's understanding of public psychiatry will deepen in the course of ensuing discussion and set a stage for consideration of the future challenges in the field. Chapter 8, the final chapter, returns to this definition, refines it, and argues that public psychiatry is a subspecialty of the larger field of general psychiatry (Brown et al., 1993; Yedida et al., 2006; Ranz et al., 2008).

To some extent, the professionals who work in the field of public psychiatry define it. Public psychiatrists follow various paths into the field of public psychiatry. These include the wish to serve particular ethnic groups, philosophical convictions about human liberation, political convictions about empowerment, beliefs about the social nature of psychiatric disorders, or a reaction to the prevailing professional ideology of the time, whether psychoanalytic or biologic. In 1963, many adherents to the new community psychiatry came from the field of social psychiatry, a subspecialty that had its own journal and advocated for attention to the family, the social environment, and nontraditional, family, and group therapies. Some psychiatrists are deeply interested in cross-cultural challenges or global mental health, both of which are prominent in pubic practice. Some psychiatrists just want to diversify their practice, which is a trend in more recent years as a growing percentage of psychiatrists work at least part time in the public sector (Ranz et al., 2006). Some psychiatrists, interested in the social sciences of epidemiology or sociology, build academic careers by linking these fields of study to public psychiatry. All these motivations and origins remain active for young psychiatric professionals who choose public psychiatry as a career.

MENTAL HEALTH AND PUBLIC HEALTH

Inherent in the definition above is the idea that public psychiatry is indeed public health psychiatry, though this is not widely appreciated in the field. In the clinical domain, the role of public psychiatry is analogous to the role of federally qualified, community health centers (CHCs) in medicine. The major difference between psychiatry and medicine is the long history of special state funding of public services for people with serious mental illness. This fact has led to the development of large state agencies, which have no counterpart in general medicine, and which manage state budgets and services. At present, the state's role is diminishing as a result of mainstreaming of mental health services and social benefits. Mainstreaming, discussed further in chapters 2 and 6, is associated with the rise of state Medicaid agencies as major players for mental health, corresponding to their role for general medicine.

Mental health, as a term, though used loosely in a variety of contexts, is the analog of public health. This assertion is an important building block in the point of view developed in this book. It is consistent with a recent publication, by the administrator of the Substance Abuse Mental Health Services Administration, about the need for public psychiatry to regain a public health perspective (Power, 2009). Undoubtedly, clinical science is a foundation of public psychiatry when clinicians offer direct service to individuals. Equally important is psychiatric epidemiologic and services research data in order for public psychiatry to understand community needs and to plan services for the populations served. What is true for public psychiatry is also true for community medicine, which makes a public health perspective essential to both.

Public psychiatry is different from medicine and public health medicine in many ways, too. However, that is not a good starting point for undertaking integration of the two, a major contemporary task. Integration appeared as a theme in public psychiatry as a function of mainstreaming, which has been a dominant mental health policy goal for over two decades. Starting with Medicaid benefits for people with serious mental illness after the repeal of the Mental Health Systems Act in 1981, mainstreaming has only intensified subsequent to the health care reform debate of 1993, the New Freedom Commission report of 2003, the documentation of the shortened life expectancy of people with serious mental illness in 2006, and health care reform in 2010.

THE PERSON WITH SERIOUS MENTAL ILLNESS

The term serious mental illness was coined to denote the most severe, recurrent, chronic or persistent disabling illnesses. It is used interchangeably in this text with the term severe and persistent mental illness, which originated in studies done at the CMHC. In epidemiologic studies, which estimate 26% of the American population suffer from mental illness, it was useful to differentiate people with the most serious psychiatric illnesses (about 6%) from those with less severe and more transient illness (about 20%). The term serious mental illness has become shorthand for people with severe, persistent schizophrenic illness; intractable bipolar illness; recurrent, unremitting depressions; intense, chronic anxiety disorders; and long-standing, incapacitating addictions. These disorders are the most profound, unrelenting, or at best intermittent, disturbances in three domains: thinking, mood, or nervousness. Often, people with serious mental illness have combinations of all three. Root causes for serious mental illnesses are unknown. While evidence-based treatments relieve symptoms, cures are not achievable. Estimates of shortened life expectancy or years lost to disability from serious mental illnesses, known as burden of disease, place them among the top ten of all kinds of diseases. As the Mental Health Services Act of 1980 asserted,

> Seriously ill psychiatric patients in the public sector are the most needy and vulnerable.

seriously ill psychiatric patients in the public sector are the most needy and vulnerable of all the patients served by psychiatry and medicine.

Most people with serious mental illness are seen in the public sector of psychiatry. For a person with serious mental illness, the pathway into the public sector varies by the nature of the illness, the course of illness over time, and access to care. Examples include young people who are no longer eligible for the health insurance of their parents. Or, caps on insurance benefits may leave a person without coverage for a chronic condition. Also, many people are incapacitated and unemployed, making employer-based insurance inaccessible. Many poor people are eligible for Medicaid, and once the illness is chronic, for Medicare. These two federal entitlements are among the main payers for services in the public sector of psychiatry. In addition, state general funds are expended through state owned services or state-administered general assistance to provide services to many uninsured. Finally, many people with serious mental illness are identified primarily, at least at first, by a major social problem they confront, whether it is homelessness, of which about 40% are considered mentally ill, or people transitioning out of prisons, of which about 80% are estimated to have addictions.

To illustrate the evolution of mental health services for people with serious mental illness, chapters 4 through 7 introduce case examples of people with serious mental illness. The "cases" are actually composites of more than one person. They are disguised to protect confidentiality of the individuals.

THE CONNECTICUT MENTAL HEALTH CENTER IN THE CONTEXT OF MODERN PUBLIC PSYCHIATRY

For more than 50 years, since deinstitutionalization began in the second half of the twentieth century, multiple strategies—organized in this book by the four periods of modern public psychiatry—have been pursued to offer effective services in the community to people with serious mental illness. The development of community services and systems is still incomplete for meeting all the needs of this target population. Each period of modern public psychiatry has made a contribution to the system, but none alone has comprehensively met the need. It is the accumulation of the innovations since the middle of the last century that approximate a complete system. In the broadest sense, this book is organized to describe and portray these service changes in modern public psychiatry at an academic community mental health center. The existing system of services now faces the challenges of yet another period of change, which is discussed in the final chapter.

After this introductory chapter, chapter 2 provides a brief overview of community and public psychiatry in the modern era since 1963. The modern era can be seen as a process of progressive deinstitutionalization from state hospitals of people with serious mental illness. As has been stated, the modern era can be broken down into four main periods: community mental health; community services and systems building; mainstreaming, and transformation. Chapter 2 considers alternate concepts, such as scientific progress and recovery, as major themes in public practice, especially during the last two periods. Also, the chapter discusses the importance of politics and economics in the shaping and changing of the field of public psychiatry. The chapter creates a context for the story of the Connecticut Mental Health Center over the modern era.

Chapter 3 introduces the services and academic programs of the CMHC. It describes the Connecticut Department of Mental Health and Addiction Services (DMHAS) and the Yale Department of Psychiatry (YDP), the two entities that are partners in the institution of the CMHC. For the YDP, a commitment to academic missions needs to accommodate the need to provide services. Sometimes academic orthodoxy, first about psychoanalysis and later biological psychiatry, has inhibited development of clinical services at the CMHC. What was lacking was a deep appreciation of the task of caring for people with serious mental illness. In the DMHAS, skepticism of academic missions runs deep, especially in times of fiscal austerity. Misunderstanding of the endowment of Yale University is rampant. For these parent entities, the CMHC is a partnership. For those who work at the CMHC, the challenge is to be part of both entities and to operationally integrate them day by day. Being part of both institutions is an essential aspect of the character of the CMHC as an institution and an essential task of management.

Chapter 4 describes the development of the CMHC, beginning when it opened in 1966, up to 1982, during the community mental health movement. Plans to establish the CMHC started in 1957 in discussions between the YDP and the state. As a result of the federal Community Mental Health Center Construction Act of 1965, the Hill West Haven (HWH) Division, which was a federally funded community mental health center, became a division of the larger institution. The remaining services of the CMHC, which were state funded, were called the General Clinical Division. In both divisions, the tension between service and academic missions played out. In 1970, the director of the CMHC resolved the conflict between state and university missions with a compromise that endured for over a decade. Through the Hill West Haven Division, federal policies largely overshadowed the state agenda until 1982. The HWH division became a model for services both at the CMHC and in the state. The rest of the CMHC slowly but progressively changed to resemble it. The novel elements of service developed during this period were the establishment of services in the community, expansion of access, timely intervention, and continuity of care.

Chapter 4 introduces a table of services developed in the period of community mental health for people with serious mental illness. It also introduces the use of case examples to illustrate service development. Each period of modern public psychiatry is associated with important contributions to the service system. Subsequent chapters return to the table to illustrate these developments. It has taken 47 years to develop the present array of services for severe mental illness. The current array of services is broad and addresses most of the needs of patients at different times in the course of illness episodes.

Chapter 5 reviews the period at the CMHC during the years of community services and system development for people with serious mental illness. It includes a discussion of community support programs and the rise again of state mental health authorities as the dominant agents for shaping policy and change. During this period, tension at the CMHC between the services and academic missions came to a head once more. Also, a crisis in leadership occurred, which had profound consequences for the CMHC and echoed for years both in the YDP and the DMHAS. Subsequently, there was a need to restore the integrity of the institution, its management, and the partnership. It was a time when regional management of services emerged, leading to the development of local mental health authorities in Connecticut. Essential service elements such as assertive community treatment (ACT,) case management, and community-based rehab services were introduced.

Chapter 6 covers a period of national mainstreaming of mental health and social welfare benefits. Mainstreaming is the alternative to the "exceptionalism" of special facility and community services development of the previous two periods (Frank and Glied, 2006). Mainstreaming on the ground in the public sector manifested itself in its handmaiden, managed care, a management tool of payers to reallocate costs, such as from expensive hospitalizations to ambulatory care, and to keep costs of medical care down. At the same time, there was a threat of privatization under a conservative Republican governor of Connecticut. The times required attention to Medicaid as a payer of services and, consequently, to the rise of state Medicaid agencies as policy makers. Within the YDP, which was progressively biological and research-oriented, it was important for the CMHC to represent the clinical mission of its faculty/staff and to support career development of clinician educators. With regard to the DMHAS, it was a time for the CMHC to renew and strengthen the connection between academic programs and the state mission of providing services, by making the academic programs indispensable in solving state policy, budgetary, and clinical challenges. Over the course of this period, academic programs such as forensic psychiatry and substance abuse, which had been growing for 25 years, became centerpieces of the CMHC portfolio. New academic programs emerged in recovery, including peer services, and medical psychiatry for integrating mental health and primary care. Service additions at the CMHC in this period included consolidation of service system elements begun in the previous period, introduction of outreach to homeless, and enhancements of primary care and wellness.

Chapter 7 addresses a period, which, while an outgrowth of mainstreaming, was shaped by the 2003 report of the President's New Freedom Commission (NFC) on Mental Health (President's NFC on Mental Health, 2003). The NFC report, building on the Surgeon General's 1999 report on mental health, recommended a transformation of the public service system. As a result of new, public health data on the shortened life expectancy of people with serious mental illness, the transformation agenda emphasized, as a central feature, integration of mental health and primary care. Also, the agenda included recovery, consumerism, person-centered care (rather than a procrustean prescription for everyone), and person-centered planning of care. At the same time, the challenges for public psychiatry expanded to include disaster readiness after the terrorist attacks of September 11, 2001. In addition, forensic community services appeared in response to the growing number of people exiting prisons on parole or termination of their sentences. All these developments diffused focus on people with serious mental illness. Recovery perspectives and peer services, such as educational and coaching programs offered by people in the process of recovery, were added to the array of services for people with serious mental illness at the CMHC.

Chapter 8 contends the present time is a critical one in the history of modern public psychiatry. The passage of health insurance parity in

2008 (Health Insurance Parity Act, 2008; Medicare Improvement Act, 2008) and health care reform in 2010 (PPAC, 2010), on top of a still-active transformation agenda from the NFC of 2003, potentially opens up a new period in modern public psychiatry. The array of services for people with serious mental illness, which is a product of development over the modern era of public psychiatry, is not secure. This chapter discusses several variables that are drivers of change in contemporary public psychiatry. These include elements of health care reform; enactment of parity in psychiatric health insurance benefits; ongoing tasks from the transformation agenda; and social, political and economic variables. The discussion emphasizes the importance of maintaining a focus on care of individuals with serious mental illness, and it indicates three contemporary themes that serve to sustain such attention. In addition to the future of public psychiatry, the chapter also considers the future of the CMHC, as a state owned, academic institution for public psychiatry. It makes the case for the academic missions of education and study in the two worlds of the academy and the public domain of the state. It concludes that academic programs at the CMHC offer forward-looking contributions to the public mission in Connecticut and the country (Jacobs and Griffith, 2007).

As a final note on the content of the book, it is important to clarify a convention used in citing names of individuals who work at the CMHC. As a general rule, the many individuals who have contributed to the evolution of the institution are not mentioned by name. It would be tedious for the general reader and would run the risk of serious omissions. The text makes sparing use of names of key leaders, who are identified with major periods of development or who initiated or headed key programs. In every case, these named individuals have had many colleagues and collaborators. It is important to acknowledge that all the developments over the years at the CMHC are the product of multiple talented and committed people. A companion volume, entitled 40 Years of Academic Psychiatry, documents many of the names and their contributions through the academic programs of the CMHC (Jacobs and Griffith, 2007).

> All the developments over the years at the CMHC are the product of multiple talented and committed people.

POINT OF VIEW

This book is a personal account of the CMHC and its history in the context of modern mental health policy. The author draws on conversations with most of the principal leaders of the institution over its lifetime, and his point of view is professional, managerial, and academic. The author started as an entry-level public health psychiatrist on an inpatient unit at the CMHC and ended as the chief executive of the institution, with a joint, academic appointment in psychiatry and public health, with both a clinical and a population perspective on mental illnesses, and with an enduring interest in evolving ideas about community mental health services. Latent in the author's judgments and opinions about the history of CMHC is a story of personal and professional development closely tied to the evolution of the institution.

The point of view is not top-down, such as that of a policy maker in Hartford, Connecticut, or Washington, D.C., nor bottom up, such as the view of a person receiving care. Nor is it primarily a view from a frontline clinician delivering the basic, mental health service, although that was a starting point for the author. Rather, the point of view is at the hub, between these two ends of the spectrum. It is the perspective from where federal and state policy and the needs of people with serious mental illness—as well as the demands of their political and community representatives—meet. For example, take the issue of managed care in public psychiatry. Managed care is a mixed blessing with respect to the basic task of obtaining or delivering services. Too often, managed care is simply a strategy used by agents of payers for the purpose rationing services and cutting costs via the inconveniences of requiring administrative approval of medical procedures ("utilization management"). Managed care also incurs high administrative costs (the "medical loss ratio"), limiting the clinical application of financial resources earmarked for patient services. Arguably, managed rationing of care deprives needed treatments to patients in some cases. On the other hand, managed care has been used effectively to reallocate resources in reified systems (such as from expensive hospital care in state systems to less expensive community care), and to control pernicious incentives for clinicians to provide quantity not quality, inherent in fee-for-service reimbursement. Also, on a social policy level, by demonstrating it could control costs managed care enabled Congressional enactment of parity of health insurance coverage for psychiatric disorders in 2008, a signal achievement for all members of American society. In sum, this book will acknowledge the value of managed care on a policy level, while addressing problems it causes in clinical practice.

The text reflects an understanding of mental health policy and an interpretation of policies in terms of their effect on the ground in one particular academic community mental health center. The point of view is not an outsider's perspective. The choice of the title, Inside Public Psychiatry is consistent with this point of view.

CONCLUSION

Public psychiatry is defined by a variety of factors, including historical development, policy statements on missions and strategy, descriptions of who public psychiatrists are and what they do, the characteristics of the populations served, and the locations where public psychiatrists work. For the purposes of this book, this introduction offers a definition, rooted in the professional literature and related to experience at the Connecticut Mental Health Center, a state owned, academic community mental health center. This is an account, since 1966, of the CMHC, which has grown as an institution during the modern era of public psychiatry—an account that illustrates most of its challenges and dilemmas. As a context for the life of this unique institution, the narrative includes a history of modern mental health policy and practice in public psychiatry. Further, the text works toward consideration of future directions in public psychiatry.

While the companion volume, 40 Years of Public Psychiatry (Jacobs and Griffith, 2007), offers a historical account of the major academic programs of the CMHC, the focus of the present book is the development of services in the context of changing mental health policies. Sometimes academic innovations have set the stage for service development and implementation in the institution. In other cases, academic programs have held back the development of services and systems. Chapter 3 discusses the relationships among the tri-partite mission of services, teaching, and research, which is part of the essential character of the CMHC.

A Brief History of Modern Public Psychiatry

Public psychiatry has a long history, beginning in the mid-nineteenth century when, as part of an international "moral treatment" movement in psychiatry, New England states began to build public hospitals to care for patients unable to afford privately financed care. Since then, the history of public psychiatry reveals a cyclical quality of optimism and pessimism, crusades and neglect, and vacillation (if not conflict) between state and federal government initiatives.

What were the policy movements that propelled the modern era and changed it over time? What new services and treatments were introduced? What problems were encountered and solutions arrived at as public psychiatry evolved? How did modern developments lead to the present? By providing an overview of the evolution of mental health policy in the modern era, this chapter begins to answer these questions. It creates a context for the story of the Connecticut Mental Health Center's history since 1966, which unfolds in the next four chapters. The abstract discussion in this chapter is illustrated by the concrete case example of this particular institution.

PERIODS IN THE MODERN ERA OF PUBLIC PSYCHIATRY

The modern era of public psychiatry can be seen as a progressive dialectic in response to the challenge to develop community services in order to cope with the deinstitutionalization of patients from state mental hospitals (see the figure in chapter 1). The modern era breaks down into four main periods (Table 2-1). There is considerable overlap among the periods. Each sows the seeds of the succeeding one.

The modern era of public psychiatry opened after the post–World War II years leading up to 1963, when Congress enacted the Community Mental Health Centers Act. The federally initiated, community mental health movement, which spawned community psychiatry as a special area of psychiatric practice, was predicated on public health concepts of

Table 2-1 Modern Periods of Mental Health Policy: Problems, Goals, and Background

Period Years	CMH 1968-82	CSSD 1982-93	Main 1993-2003	Trans 2003-10	Reform 2010-
Problems	Chronic care and overcrowding in psychiatric hospitals	Inadequate services for SPMI in community	Discriminatory health insurance for mental illness	Fragmented service system, inadequate funding	Uninsured people
Goals	De-institutionalization, community treatment, and PH interventions	Rehab services, housing, and social supports	Evidence for efficacy of psychiatric treatment to achieve parity	Transformation of MH "system," state by state, recovery as a theme	Access to care through health insurance
Underlying politics and economics	Post-WW II federal activism, federal funding, initiative falls short during economic recessions of the 1970s	Repeal of MHSA in 81, reaganomics, state DMHs lead, Medicaid rises as a payer	Clinton supports parity, SG report on MH, economic cycles strain MH budgets	Neo-conservative economics, new federalism, state initiative, and private ownership	Slow recovery from 2008 recession, increased demand/cost concerns
Other themes and issues	Both clinical and political goals, social optimism, psychoanalytic therapies prevail in 1960s, DSM-III in 1980	Political skepticism about the role of government, biological psychiatry rises	Health insurance reform debate in 1993 focuses psychiatry on parity	MH system repudiated, MH parity in 208 nursing homes D/C MH patients, integrated MH and primary care	Patient-centered, medical homes, chronic disease programs

early intervention, treatment in the community, and continuity of care (Foley and Sharfstein, 1983).

The second period began in 1982 after the Reagan administration repealed the Mental Health Systems Act (MHSA) enacted in 1980 under the Carter administration. Though the sweeping recommendations of President Jimmy Carter's presidential Commission on Mental Health for expansion of the national community mental health system were rejected, a policy focus on people with serious mental illness and many innovative ideas survived in a National Plan for the Chronically Mentally Ill, published by the National Institute of Mental Health (USDHHS, 1980). Policy initiatives on a federal level became piecemeal (Grob and Goldman, 2007). Under a renewed federalism, it was a time when states, through their departments of mental health, led local communities in the development of community services and systems.

The third period, which began in 1993, was one of mainstreaming mental health and social benefits into existing federal entitlements and welfare programs (Frank and Glied, 2006). Beginning during the previous decade, success in passing Medicaid legislation to build reimbursement for essential community-based services for people with serious mental illness was a harbinger of mainstreaming (Grob and Goldman, 2007). As a corollary, states pursued federal Medicaid matching funds—the Federal Medicaid Assistance Percentage (FMAP)—in order to ease their fiscal crises. The logic was simple: If states could manage and control the volume of services, they could reduce their expenditures by 50% or more. Mainstreaming, first of Medicaid mental health benefits, then of all mental health insurance benefits, was an alternative to the 1982 repeal of the Carter administration's MHSA, which proposed a national system of special services for people with serious mental illness. However, mainstreaming also was an expression of policy strategies that emerged from the national health care debate of 1993, when it became apparent that psychiatric services needed to integrate with medicine in order to achieve the benefits of universal health insurance and to end discriminatory health insurance benefits for behavioral disorders.

Transformation was the fourth period, which began in 2003. It was an outgrowth of mainstreaming, launched by a report of the New Freedom Commission during the Bush administration (President's New Freedom Commission on Mental Health, 2003). During transformation, attention shifted to integration of mental health into primary care, integration of mental health and substance-abuse services, and recovery from illness.

It is possible that a new period of public psychiatry is opening as a result of implementation of parity of psychiatric insurance benefits (Health Insurance Parity, 2008; Medicare Improvement Act, 2008) and the enactment of health care reform in 2010 (PPAC Act, 2010). Both expand access to mental health insurance. The implementation timetable of health care reform is nine years. Chapters 7 and 8 speculate on the possibilities of these major policy landmarks for the future of public psychiatry.

EARLY HISTORY OF PUBLIC PSYCHIATRY

The origins of public psychiatry can be traced to Dorothea Dix and the nineteenth-century American movement to bring the benefits of moral psychiatry to a wider public. Originating in Europe, the moral psychiatry movement had been responsible for the opening of private institutes such as Friend's Hospital in Philadelphia and the Institute of Living in Hartford, Connecticut. Moral treatment was predicated on separating psychiatric patients from jailed criminals and providing care for them in separate institutions. These new institutions offered moral education, cultural experiences, and a safe, supportive environment, not to mention some idiosyncratic treatments for recovery from mental illnesses. Dix had been successful in persuading many states to open public psychiatric hospitals. In 1854, President Franklin Pierce vetoed legislation passed by Congress in response to Dix's pleas. This failed legislation would have created a federal role in caring for patients with serous mental illness. The veto left responsibility for the indigent mentally ill in the hands of the states and local communities.

Over the next 50 years, states opened large, publicly funded hospitals that became known as asylums. The State of Connecticut constructed Connecticut Valley Hospital and eventually four other state owned and operated hospitals. These state hospitals, which complemented privately operated hospitals, became the cornerstones of public sector psychiatry and care. The absence of effective treatments, the chronic nature of serious psychiatric disorders, the difficulty of discharging symptomatic patients back into the community, and eventual overcrowding compromised quality of care in the public sector. Accordingly, this sector of mental health services went through cyclical periods of deprivation and optimistic renewal. In the circumstances of long-term hospital care in large state facilities in the early twentieth century, the mental hygiene movement emerged, promoting early intervention and community clinics. Its champion was Clifford Beers, a Yale College graduate, who suffered from bipolar disorder and had been hospitalized at Connecticut Valley Hospital for over a year.

The introduction of mental hygiene clinics, especially for children, heralded an ambulatory capacity for psychiatric practice to supplement the large, established psychiatric hospitals. The majority of psychiatric practice occurred in the public sector of psychiatric hospitals or in budding academic departments of psychiatry. Typically, the general adult public continued to receive care in the public system and in the hospital.

THE POST–WORLD WAR II PERIOD
IN PUBLIC PSYCHIATRY

In the post–World War II period there occurred a major reaction to custodial and, often, poor quality care of patients in large state hospitals. It culminated in federal enactment of Community Mental Health Act in 1963, which launched the community mental health movement (Grob, 1991). In the 1948 Public Health Service Act, the federal government, had created the NIMH. The National Mental Illness and Health Act of 1955 stimulated the development of state mental health authorities (state departments of mental health) that were intended to pick up the costs and management of community care as an alternative to the old state hospitals (Foley and Sharfstein, 1983). In addition the NIMH stimulated the development of outpatient clinics for follow up of patients discharged from the hospital. As a result of these initiatives, the public sector of psychiatry featured newly created mental health authorities and large state hospitals, which were still the foundation of the system, as well as a growing number of outpatient clinics linked to the hospitals. In 1961, shortly after the Kennedy administration took office, a congressional joint commission created by the Mental Illness and Health Act of 1955 issued a report entitled "Action for Mental Health." Professional, political and economic forces were aligned, creating a situation ripe for reform.

The community mental health movement, which blossomed after 1963, was a product of many contributing factors. These included wartime lessons in early intervention, the emergence of new treatments such as the antipsychotic drug, chlorpromazine, and considerable therapeutic optimism rooted in part in psychoanalytic theory. It is important to note other key developments, which coincidentally came in 1963 with, or shortly after, the Community Mental Health Centers Act. One development was an expansion in the role of general hospitals in the acute care of psychiatric patients. Also, reimbursement by Medicaid and Medicare, both enacted in 1965, funded the alternative hospital services in general hospitals and accelerated deinstitutionalization from the large state hospitals. Medicaid and the Social Security Act of 1965, which established disability insurance, enabled the expansion of nursing homes throughout the United States. Nursing homes became a decentralized, largely "invisible" destination for trans-institutionalization of chronically ill patients in state psychiatric hospitals. The general hospitals and nursing homes became major building blocks in a modern system of care for patients treated in the community and in the public sector.

THE COMMUNITY MENTAL HEALTH MOVEMENT, 1963–82

After John F. Kennedy's election in 1960, a presidential task force soon began consideration of federal, community mental health policy (Grob, 1991; Foley and Sharfstein, 1983). In 1963, following recommendations of the task force, which largely ignored the 1955 Joint Commission on Mental Illness and Health, President Kennedy sent a message to Congress calling for "a bold new approach" to mental health, and for mentally ill people "to be successfully and quickly treated in their own communities and returned to a useful place in society." The Community Mental Health Centers Act set a goal "to retain in and to return to the community the mentally ill and there to restore and revitalize their lives through better health programs and strengthened educational and rehabilitation services, and to reinforce the will and capacity of our communities to meet these programs." Community mental health was part of a larger, optimistic social movement of this time in American society. During President Lyndon B. Johnson's administration, this social movement became known as a war on poverty. The community mental health movement was national in scope, occurring in reaction to the perceived ills of large state hospitals. It included faith in the efficacy of modern psychiatry and concern for social justice, even as skeptics criticized its lofty, untested goals.

The head of the NIMH advanced the idea of local centers, instead of clinics. The plan was for these centers to have active involvement in the community. The centers would be located in defined geographic areas called "catchments." They were intended to provide coordinated and continuous services to mentally ill patients where they lived, thereby addressing a fragmented conglomeration of separate, independent hospitals, clinics, and agencies that served people with psychiatric disorders. The themes of coordination, and eventually integration, in response to the seemingly intractable fragmentation of mental health services, continued unabated through the modern era. Based on public health concepts of primary, secondary, and tertiary prevention, the services offered by the centers included early identification of disease and prevention through taking action on social stresses and other environmental etiologies as part of programs including five essential services.

During the next 17 years federal policy initiatives and, starting in 1965, the massive investment in the construction and staffing of community mental health centers eclipsed traditional state mental health authorities and their institutions. The novel community mental health centers began to open in 1966. By 1978, there were 675 fully funded community mental health centers across the United States (Foley and Sharfstein, 1983). Although this construction feat was quite an achievement, more than 800 unfunded catchment areas remained without federally funded operational centers, in part as a result of budget constraints created by the cost of the Vietnam War. The community mental health movement and the construction of community mental health centers occurred in the circumstances of accelerating release of patients from state psychiatric hospitals across the nation (see the figure in chapter 1).

Community mental health centers, though falling short in their attention to the most chronically ill, played an important role in deinstitutionalization—along with the enactment of federal entitlements, the rise of nursing homes, and progressive development of patient rights. In 1977, community mental health centers served almost two million people, including many representatives of ethnic and racial minorities and previously underserved people in rural areas (Foley and Sharfstein, 1983). After eight years, federal dollars were being matched by state and private dollars on a four to one basis. There was enormous development in the scope and diversity of treatments available in the community. Indeed, community mental health centers reduced admissions to state hospitals in areas where they were co-located. Between 1955 and 1977 the number of patient-care episodes (mostly admissions) in state hospitals declined from 818,000 to 574,000, while outpatient patient-care episodes went up from less than one million to 4.6 million. Psychiatric beds in state hospitals declined from 623,000 to 124,000 (see the figure in chapter 1), while beds in general hospitals and community mental health centers grew in number. Direct expenditures for mental illness went from $1.2 billion to $19.6 billion. Coincident with the rise of community mental health centers, there was a tremendous increase in the number of mental health professionals as a product of NIMH training grants. The number of psychiatrists increased from 10,600 in 1955 to more than 30,000 in 1980. Psychologists increased from 13,500 to 56,933. The number of psychiatric social workers increased the most, from 20,000 to 89,000.

Trans-institutionalization of patients in state hospitals also was an important part of these remarkable changes. During this period, there was also tremendous growth of the private nursing home industry. This growth was a result of funding provided by the federal Social Security Act of 1965 and Medicaid. From 1954 to 1973, funding grew from $170,000 to $1.4 million. State hospitals discharged patients to nursing homes, where typically a modicum of clinical followup was provided, but no true integration into the community was possible. The trans-institutionalization of patients helped masked the unfortunate failure of most community mental health centers to meet the needs of many people who had serious and persistent mental illnesses. While reaching out to new populations and providing comprehensive services in substantial ways, as noted above, the centers failed the most chronic and disabled population. This failure became a major issue for the Carter administration's presidential commission on mental health.

After President Carter's election in 1976, he formed the Presidential Commission on Mental Health, chaired by his wife, Rosalyn Carter. In 1978, the commission reported on the state of mental health services, emphasizing the deficiencies in the care of chronically ill individuals. The report suggested several strategies for improving that care. Congress enacted many of the recommendations into law in the 1980 MHSA. The MHSA affirmed a societal commitment both to community-based treatment and to support services for chronically ill, low income, mentally ill people. It also restructured federal, state, and local roles, emphasized prevention—largely through linkage to primary care—and recommended a patient bill of rights. Before these recommendations could be implemented, unfortunately, the repeal of the MHSA in 1981 by the Reagan administration marked the end of direct federal funding of community mental health centers by means of construction and staffing grants. In place of these, the Reagan administration initiated block grants to states, which served the purpose of capping federal expenditures on mental health services and reactivated the role of state mental health authorities in mental health policy and services.

Between 1963 and 1982, state departments of mental health and hospitals receded into the background of the massive federally funded, community mental health movement, while pursuing change in their own right. For them, the main challenge was progressive discharge of institutionalized patients from state hospitals. In 1982, with the end of federal, categorical funding for community mental health centers, the state mental health authorities surged into prominence again as part of a renewed, federalist philosophy. State mental health authorities, in concert with federal demonstration grants and legislative initiatives regarding Medicaid, were key players in the development of community-based services and systems for people with serious mental illness. In this way they shaped an evolving definition of public psychiatry.

COMMUNITY SERVICES AND SYSTEMS FOR PEOPLE WITH SERIOUS MENTAL ILLNESS, 1982–93

Beginning in 1982, after repeal of the MHSA and following the national Plan for the Chronically Mentally Ill published by the Surgeon General in 1980, piecemeal federal legislative initiatives continued to define the early part of this new period of community services and system development (Grob and Goldman, 2007). In this new period, Medicaid reimbursement played a critical role in supporting development of community-based services for people with serious mental illness. The rise of Medicaid as a payer reflected the importance of collaboration between federal and state authorities. Under Medicaid, states submitted plans that required review by the federal Center for Medicare and Medicaid Services to assure compliance with federal policy requirements. The types of services and parameters of service were defined by federal Medicaid regulations, even as states exercised considerable choice over the extent and shape of Medicaid programs.

As a result of a series of legislative victories over the next 10 years, Medicaid began to reimburse essential services for people with serious mental illness in the community. These included clinic-based services, case management, and psychosocial rehabilitation. As state general fund dollars diminished due to periodic state budget deficits, states and private nonprofit community mental health centers turned to Medicaid as a reimbursement for mental health services. For states, the process was known as "medicaiding" services in order to be eligible for Medicaid matching reimbursement (FMAP). Private nonprofit agencies were establishing a revenue stream that would support staff and administration. Medicaid Supplemental Security Income, by providing income supports for poor people, and Medicaid health insurance together became a foundation for community living for large numbers of low-income individuals with psychiatric disorders. By 2001, the two main payers of public services were Medicaid and state departments of behavioral services (Mark et al., 2007). Medicaid was the single largest payer. While medicaiding services was a great benefit to those who were Medicaid-eligible, it is important to note that many people were not eligible, and they had to rely on services supported by state general assistance or general fund dollars.

> By 2001, the two main payers of public services were Medicaid and state departments of behavioral services.

In response to a growing concern that chronically ill people were not well cared for by community mental health centers, the NIMH opened a Community Support Program (CSP) in 1977. NIMH created this new office for the purpose of funding demonstration projects, building a data base, and disseminating programs on "comprehensive community support systems for severely, mentally disabled adults" (Turner and Tenhoor, 1978). This program also advocated a "systems perspective as a basis for planning services." It was a strategic bridge into the new period of public psychiatry. The CSP office offered a vehicle for federal policy development through demonstration contracts with state departments of mental health on outreach and integrated community services. Dissemination of assertive community treatment and stimulation of managed service systems, eventually known as local mental health authorities, are examples of initiatives that helped shape a system of care for people with serious mental illness.

Based on a belief in the value of providing authority and accountability for system development and integration, the concept of local mental health authorities was another iteration of federal thinking about how to best implement and coordinate mental health care. Many community mental health centers, as agents of state mental health authorities, served as the new local authority. Though each state department of mental health played out its own version of this change, the movement was national in scope.

> Many community mental health centers served as the new local authority.

It is important to note in passing that the value of system efforts, when later tested by a Robert Wood Johnson study and two NIMH studies, did not prove out to enhance the quality of care and outcomes of treatment for individuals with serious mental illness.

These developments on a federal and state level focused the definition of a target population for public psychiatry. In contrast to the community mental health period, when the definition was largely a function of geographic location, the new definition of a target population focused more narrowly on people with serious mental illness. Even as this shift in definition of the target population was occurring, the focus on people with serious mental illness was decreasing as states medicaided services. The broader Medicaid-eligible population was brought under the tent of public psychiatry. From this point forward, the progressive diffusion of a narrow population targeted by public psychiatry would become a function of challenges that needed to be met over the next two decades. These included the need to address social problems such as homelessness, and the need to serve people embroiled in criminal justice systems, and also disaster readiness.

The once broad roles of community psychiatrists narrowed during this second period of modern public psychiatry. During the community mental health movement, psychiatrists played prominent roles in the early phase of policy development, in the implementation, in the management of the new centers, and as clinical team leaders. As a result of the proliferation of mental health professionals, of non-medical leadership in community mental health centers, of recurrent fiscal crises, and of the high cost of psychiatrists, psychiatrists were relegated to diminished and limited roles. It became increasingly hard to find psychiatrists in positions of institutional leadership, management, and even in clinical team leadership. Physicians largely became high-volume prescribers in systems that tended to devalue medical services and instead to emphasize rehabilitation of chronic illness. Partlyas a means of protesting this constriction of physicians' roles, the American Association of Community Psychiatrists was formed in 1984. Psychiatrists split off from community mental health in order to advocate for leadership and broad professional roles for physicians in community practice, even as they continued to embrace the basic tenets of the community mental health movement.

During this period of community services and system development, Medicaid underwrote much of the services and system development for people with serious mental illness. Before the achievement of parity of insurance benefits for federal employees in 1996, this was the leading example of mainstreaming mental health benefits in a federal entitlement program. Indeed, the overall success in obtaining Medicaid reimbursement for mental health services during this decade can be seen as a case study of mainstreaming in the public sector, which mental health advocates then generalized to all public and private payers. Thus, depending on whether one emphasizes—as an example of mainstreaming—either the role of Medicaid in support of the new community-based services or the role of Medicaid reimbursement, it is possible to bring Medicaid into the discussion in both periods: that of community services and system development and the succeeding one of mainstreaming. There is no clear end to the period of community services and system development in public psychiatry. Just as community mental health centers survived and morphed into new roles during community services development, the elements of service in the community for people with serious mental illness remained as building blocks during subsequent periods.

MAINSTREAMING OF MENTAL HEALTH SERVICES, 1993–2003

The national health care debate of 1993, during the Clinton administration, is a reasonable point in time for the identification of a new period—termed mainstreaming in public psychiatry. The national health care debate had illustrated that psychiatric services needed to identify with, if not integrate with, medicine in order to benefit from health insurance reform and end discriminatory mental health insurance benefits, which was a blight for people with psychiatric disorders. Mainstreaming refers to a period when the key mental health policy objectives turned to the integration of mental health and social welfare benefits into the mainstream of general health care and welfare programs (Frank and Glied, 2006). In a sense, mainstreaming was a reaction to the failure, at the beginning of the Reagan era, to expand the community mental health movement and create a national system of special services for people with serious mental illness. In contrast to the sweeping system changes recommended in the MHSA of 1980, legislative initiatives going forward were parsed, sequential, and aimed at particular entitlement, insurance, and welfare programs, and were pursued with an eye on the ultimate goal of parity of health insurance coverage for people with psychiatric disorders.

State departments of mental health transitioned from their role as providers of service in state owned facilities to the role of purchasers of service from private, nonprofit agencies in the community. This process was driven by economic recessions and state budget deficits in 1980-81, 1990-91, and 2001-02. Private, nonprofit agencies grew as a result of this process. Also, when state Medicaid agencies began to contract with private behavioral managed care organizations, a reduction of the influence of state mental health authorities became apparent. Tracing the evolution of state general fund budgets for mental health starting in 1980, a shift occurred. State general fund support for state hospitals, which closed over time, shifted to ambulatory services. State-provided ambulatory services were replaced by services purchased and provided in the community by private, nonprofit agencies. In this way, similar to the effects of the introduction of Medicaid and Medicare in 1965, the boundaries and distinctions between public and private sector services blurred, making it difficult to discern when, during patients' careers in treatment, they were in the private or public domain.

In 1996, a Clinton White House conference on mental health signaled that mainstreaming had matured and promised to deliver substantial and tangible results. It was at this conference that President Clinton announced parity of health insurance coverage for mental disorders under federal employee health insurance plans. This achievement was a milestone. It was a forerunner to parity under Medicare and commercial plans enacted in 2008 and health care reform in 2010, which ratified parity in the health insurance benefits extended to the uninsured.

The White House conference of 1996 was a prelude to a 1999 report on mental health by the Surgeon General of the United States, the first ever of its kind. In rapid succession, two other reports appeared about suicide and disparities in mental health care outcomes. These reports set a new course for mental health and addiction services in the public sector. It was yet another manifestation of mainstreaming. The surgeon general's Report on Mental Health endorsed the idea of mainstreaming mental health with general health and welfare policy and noted substantial progress in establishing the efficacy of psychiatric treatments (U.S. Department of Health and Human Services, 1999). The report concluded that services were provided in a "de facto," non-system that had grown as new mental health initiatives sprouted over the years. Further, the report recommended a major goal of implementing evidence-based practice throughout the system in order to deliver effective treatments to the public. Two years later, in 2001, the surgeon general issued a call to action to reduce suicides, thereby providing the first national public health message on a major source of mortality from psychiatric disorders (U.S. Department of Health and Human Services, 2001). In another report the same year, the surgeon general directed attention to disparities in healthcare outcomes for members of minority populations and reinforced a call, from his first report, for culturally competent care (U.S. Department of Health and Human Services, 2001).

In 2001, the Institute of Medicine (IOM) published its landmark report, *Crossing the Quality Chasm* (Institute of Medicine, 2001). This report created an agenda for improving patient safety and quality of care through evidence-based practices. The Joint Commission on Accreditation of Healthcare Organizations carried this agenda forward by establishing quality-improvement and patient safety as core elements of its review criteria for periodic site visits of healthcare facilities. More than ever before, information technology now provided the tools for monitoring quality, and also made quality information available to the public via the internet. Payers, including Medicare, developed pay-for-performance strategies to create incentive for delivering optimal care.

By the turn of the century, Medicaid, a main payer of services in public psychiatry, emerged as the leading line item in many state budgets. Unfortunately this new fact came to light in the circumstances of state budget crises in the economic recession of 2001. Under these circumstances, states raised questions about limiting eligibility, restricting benefits, capping utilization, and managing utilization. Behavioral managed care companies were the agents of the states in pursuit of their cost control strategies. In addition Medic-

> In 2001 states raised questions about limiting eligibility, restricting benefits, and capping and managing utilization.

aid reform loomed on the horizon for the purpose of the federal government capping its costs and also to enable states to control theirs. A Medicaid
Reform Commission during the Bush administration did not report out
until 2007. Limits on eligibility, which would exclude individuals traditionally served by state departments of mental health, were a worry. Also
of great potential concern were limits on benefits, which would restrict
access to essential outreach and community support services needed by
chronically ill people. There were latent threats to the "optional" Medicaid
services enacted subsequent to 1982, such as case management, community support programs, and assertive community treatment.

In 2001, the Bush administration created a presidential commission on
mental health called the New Freedom Commission (NFC). This presidential commission began about a quarter of a century after the Carter
Commission. The period of mainstreaming was in full swing, with the
commission, which was a part of it, promising a fresh look at mental
health.

TRANSFORMATION, 2003–PRESENT

In 2003, under the Bush administration, the NFC on Mental Health concluded—as did the surgeon general a few years before and all commission reports since the Kennedy era—that the mental health system was
in disarray (President's NFC, 2003). The system was a "patchwork relic,"
and was "in shambles." Although unable, under a presidential stipula-
tion, to advocate for new resources to accomplish its purpose, the NFC
recommended a transformation of the system of care.

The transformation would be built upon a foundation that emphasized six fundamental goals:

(1) public education to reduce stigma and highlight the centrality of mental
     health to overall health;
(2) consumer and family driven care, with consumers in recovery and family
     fully involved in treatment planning and system development;
(3) the elimination of disparities in services through improving cultural com-
     petence and access to care;
(4) establishment of early screening, assessment, and referral as common
     practice, across the lifespan and in primary care and school settings;
(5) the delivery of excellent health care through disseminating evidence-based
     practices and accelerating research, particularly into recovery and under-
     studied areas such as trauma, acute care, and disparities in outcomes; and
(6) the use of technology to enhance access to care and to health information,
     through the development of integrated electronic, psychiatric records and
     personal health information systems.

In 2005, the Substance Abuse Mental Health Services Administration issued a so-called road map, a transformation plan for federal agencies, and awarded demonstration grants to seven states, including Connecticut. As part of the "new federalism" philosophy of the NFC, states had considerable latitude in developing local solutions within a federally defined framework. Unfortunately, states were faced with the prospect of proceeding in the circumstances of an economic crisis and severe budget constraints created, in part, by the growth of Medicaid health care costs.

The NFC report also embeds the challenge of integrating mental health and primary care under the goal of recognizing the centrality of mental health to overall health. This task became even more urgent with the growing appreciation of the shortened life expectancy of people with serious mental illness (National Association of State Mental Health Program Directors, 2006). Integration was a major building block in mainstreaming public mental health with general health and welfare policy.

There are echoes of the community mental health movement the NFC report. This is most conspicuous in the renewed focus on placing mental health care in the context of a public health agenda. Examples of a public health approach are: early intervention programs, prevention of suicide, a focus on high-risk groups such as ethnic minorities whose treatment outcomes lag, and the burden of disease from psychiatric disorders. Also, the integration of mental health and medicine, never successfully addressed during the community mental health period, referred back to that period. These were examples of how the mainstream and transformation thinking was broader than the narrow, if not exclusive, focus of the previous period. Drawing the most attention at that time was care of chronically ill individuals, which was given to continuous care, rehabilitation, and community supports. These new considerations gave impetus to a search, in public psychiatry, for a medical model broad enough to encompass an entire spectrum of services needed especially by people with serious mental illness.

ALTERNATE CHOICES FOR MAJOR FORCES SHAPING CHANGE IN PUBLIC PSYCHIATRY

While it is possible with some conviction to identify the first period of modern public psychiatry, the last three periods are more ambiguous. For example, the last two periods are still evolving—not to mention being overtaken by health care reform. More time will be needed to conclude what label best denotes them.

Three other major processes deserve consideration as forces, or variables, shaping public psychiatry since the community mental health movement ended in 1982. Each process might serve as the label for a particular period of development. They are: (a) the rise of Medicaid as a funder of services for people with serious mental illness; (b) the recovery movement for people with mental illnesses, and (c) the translation of neurobiological, psychological, and social sciences into practice. Each of the three overlaps periods used here to break down and define the modern era of public psychiatry. Medicaid spans system development and mainstreaming. Recovery spans mainstreaming and transformation. Translation spans all the periods of modern public psychiatry. After the publication of the new *Diagnostic and Statistical Manual* in 1980, momentum picked up in the scientific study of psychiatric etiology and treatment.

This chapter previously discussed the process of medicaiding services during the second and third periods, as states pursued matching federal reimbursement as an alternative to using general fund dollars. Medicaiding was most prominent in the period of community services and system development (Cutler et al., 2003). The choice of a label for that period reflected an emphasis on the community-based services that emerged, the target population of the period, and the fact that some aspects of the period such as system development were not intrinsic to Medicaid. Reasons for not choosing the other two variables as labels for periods are discussed next.

RECOVERY

The recovery movement in psychiatry aimed to empower those who suffered from mental illness, many of whom felt disenfranchised or—more ominously in terms of their attitude toward psychiatric professionals—considered themselves as survivors of psychiatric treatment. Equally important, the recovery movement instilled hope of a fuller life and membership in the community (Davidson, 2003; Davidson, et al., 2005, 2006). The movement grew over two decades and eventually was highlighted in the NFC report of 2003. The recovery movement can be understood as a culmination of the expansion of civil rights for people with mental illness. The rights of patients to treatment in psychiatric hospitals were defined in court decisions, beginning notably in the Wyatt versus Stickney Supreme Court case in 1969 (*Wyatt v. Stickney*, 1971). The National Alliance of Mentally Ill, mostly an organization of families of people with mental illness, appeared in 1979 and became a powerful voice for people with mental illnesses. The recovery movement was indigenous to psychiatry, as people with mental illness began to write about their personal experiences. Importantly, however, it was also part of a mainstream movement toward consumerism and ownership in general medicine and welfare programs. For over 30 years, people with diseases of all kinds were demanding a voice in their own care and recovery from illness. Progressively, a consumer voice in clinical care emerged at all levels of the public system.

As one might expect of a social movement of empowerment, advocates for recovery were often understandably antagonistic to the established system of care and the professionals who represent it. Even worse, mental health professionals could be seen as agents of oppression, from whom liberation was a goal. As a civil rights movement that demands attention and change, recovery upset the establishment. This may be essential to the success of a social movement, but it does not facilitate acceptance by the professionals, who work in the public domain. Most professional psychiatrists look for evidence to support the claims of advantages by recovery advocates. As a starting point, it is important to remember that some foundations of the recovery movement were rooted in modern clinical science that provided evidence of trajectories of recovery in many people with serious mental illness (Strauss et al., 1985; Harding et al., 1987). The discrepancy between rhetoric and evidence seems intrinsic to new movements in mental health. Ultimately, however, it will be evidence that carries the day in the professional world of public practice. Developing evidence takes time.

In the meantime, the recovery movement has been instrumental in giving voice to people who are mentally ill. It requires that the voice of sick people be included in public debate and in the clinical practice of those caring for them. It can play a role in improving access to, and retention in, treatment. Not surprisingly, payers and providers of service have appropriated and used recovery rhetoric for their own purposes. These include public relations efforts seeking competitive advantage in the marketplace and pursuit of cost control, by shifting responsibility and expenses from payers to consumers as part of ownership. Even though recovery is not clinical, per se, if it successfully evolves then it has the potential to transform clinical practice by incorporating people with an illness, their goals and wishes, into the clinical planning process. Person-centered care planning is an evidence-based procedure for accomplishing this goal. As such, it is one, but only one, of several transformational themes that ought to be included in any consideration of the transformation period. On the other hand, until the recovery movement demonstrates its effectiveness by the accumulation of evidence, it does not warrant top billing as the keynote of a period.

TRANSLATION

Translation is another theme of the past several years that merits consideration as a major force changing contemporary public psychiatry (Drake et al., 2003). Translation is the process of introducing scientific discoveries into practice. With the 1980 publication of the *Diagnostic and Statistical Manual*, Version III, which defined the terms of psychiatric disorders, clinical psychiatry—while already building a scientific base—was poised to enter a scientific renaissance. Indeed, much has been accomplished, as documented in the 1999 surgeon general's report. While progress in psychosocial treatments (such as therapies codified in manuals) and rehabilitation interventions (such as social and work skills training), little progress has been made in pharmacologic treatments. Despite the "decade of the brain" and pharmaceutical company hyperbole, psychopharmacology has not substantially progressed. The CATIE study demonstrated this state of affairs for antipsychotic drugs (Lieberman et al., 2005). Psychiatrists have more drugs to choose from in treating mental illnesses, which facilitates finding the optimal benefit-to-side effect ratio for individual patients. Nevertheless, lacking in the past 40 years is any fundamental discovery about the nature of psychiatric disorders or any breakthroughs in treatment of people with serious mental illness, the core group served by public psychiatry.

Public psychiatry in the past decade has witnessed a series of landmark reports that, while documenting the evidence base for modern psychiatric practice, reach troubling conclusions. While the report of the surgeon general documented the evidence for psychiatric treatments, it contained ominous notes on delays and deficiencies in adopting evidence-based practices, i.e., inadequate translation, and on the existence of cross-cultural disparities in outcomes. Also, the report concluded that the system of care was a de facto hodgepodge of services that were fragmented and poorly coordinated, handicapping the delivery of care. The presidential New Freedom Commission report of 2003 reinforced this conclusion.

Another major overview of mental health over the last half of the twentieth century, entitled *Better But Not Well*, documented progress in the number of people having access to psychiatric treatment and mainstream social benefits (Frank and Glied, 2006). It concluded that most of that progress in the status of people with serious mental illness came not from diagnostic or treatment advances but rather from improvement of access to existing treatment

> Most progress came not from diagnostic or treatment advances but from improvement of access.

and social welfare benefits. The authors concluded that people with serious mental illness were "better but not well," prompting the title of their book. An update in 2009 suggested continuing cause for concern about the most recent years (Glied and Frank, 2009). Access for seniors with mental illness was dropping and the allocation of expenditures for drugs was soaring—despite the absence of evidence to prove the new treatments were superior.

The NFC report stimulated a comprehensive and fundamental review of federally funded mental health research by NIMH. Published in 2009, the broad conclusions of the review about progress in psychiatric research were discouraging. Using public health data, the NIMH report concluded that no reduction in prevalence of major mental disorders had occurred in the past 50 years and that the advances made in the understanding of psychiatric disorders and their treatment were modest at best. Little or no improvement was discernable in recovery or in the reduction of burden in disease. The lag of development in psychiatric research stood in contrast to other fields of medicine, such as cardiology and oncology, where by the same metrics progress was observable. Further, major breakthroughs in genomic research were neither imminent nor probable using research strategies employed over the past 10 years. The NIMH report concluded that the biological models of the past 50 years, based on symptoms and descriptive diagnostic categories and on a time-honored focus on drug development strategies, were dead ends. Though a source of powerful promise, and a method for progress rather than cyclical, ideological dialectics, translation of mental health research and its discoveries into practice does not measure up as a major force, especially in regard to the main charge of public psychiatry, which is caring for people with serious mental illness.

SUMMARY OF MEDICAID, RECOVERY, AND TRANSLATION AS FACTORS IN MODERN PUBLIC PSYCHIATRY

In summary, recovery's impact on practice is still unproven, and it is just one of many important goals under transformation. Translation, despite its contributions to quality and effectiveness of care, simply has not risen to prominence as a major force for change, despite a fundamental conviction that science will lead the way to a new future in psychiatric practice. Both recovery and translation span long periods of time and offer less opportunity for discrimination and differentiation in thinking about modern public psychiatry. Medicaid policies are also forces shaping modern public psychiatry that spans three periods of development, since 1982. Medicaid is a powerful undercurrent that operates more subtly and remains quite active and will play a key role in extending health insurance benefits under health care reform. The importance of Medicaid—or, in the broadest sense, of the budgeting and financing of services—leads to the next section on the politics and economics of public psychiatry.

POLITICS, ECONOMICS, AND PUBLIC PSYCHIATRY

In 1973, at a time of ferment over the future of public psychiatry, the director of the CMHC wrote a paper that emphasized the "pragmatics" of community mental health care (Astrachan, 1974). The paper put forward the proposition that, as forces shaping change, politics and economics trumped professional, scientific, and ideological considerations. Often, politics and economics conflate into what the paper called "politico-economics," as, for example, when elected state executives are faced with severe budget deficits. Over the modern era of public psychiatry there have been several major economic recessions—1973, 1982, 1991, 2001, and 2008. These recessions have often served as critical points at which the system lurched in a new direction. For example, the Reagan administration policies, intended to control health care costs by using good business practice and economic incentives, rendered the economic side of politico-economics even more important, not to mention the importance of the political philosophy of federalism. It was a landmark of the Reagan era when corporate and business cultures were introduced into medicine, challenging a clinical approach that had prevailed until that time.

This book espouses the view that federal and state fiscal crises and mechanisms of financing care (benefit eligibility, benefit package definition, reimbursement policies, utilization management) are the bridge between policy and practice. Understanding financing mechanisms and utilization management by payers is a key to understanding how the system works. A powerful way to track the vicissitudes and future directions of public psychiatry is to "follow the money." to borrow a term from the Watergate era. This point of view is based on an existential logic that goes like this: Professionals are defined by what they do. They do what they are paid for. Payers and their reimbursement policies largely define what professionals do. In other words, reimbursement shapes the system in which clinicians work, the things clinicians do, and their identity as clinicians. For example, since 1990, the intrusion of managed care into the practice of long-term psychotherapy by psychiatrists who believed they were entitled to higher fees given their special education, has transformed psychiatric practice. Younger generations of professionals are particularly sensitive to these forces. As a result, not only did the duration of psychotherapy diminish, but so did the number of hours devoted in practice to psychotherapy.

While this point of view on politico-economics undoubtedly seems cynical, it is useful for reading current and imminent change, especially when the real policy goals cannot be talked about in public for fear of hostile public reaction and political storms. The vicissitudes of funding for mental health services help explain not only the "shambles" in which the mental health system finds itself but also the need for periodic national commissions in order to renew the social commitment to caring for those with serious mental illness.

Each of the four periods of modern public psychiatry is associated with a predominant approach to funding public psychiatry. In addition, a fundamental dynamic to follow is cost shifting between federal and state governments. During the community mental health movement, as a result of public resolve to do something about the warehousing of psychiatric patients in large state hospitals, federal money poured into states and local communities. This funding bypassed state departments of mental health and went directly to grantees in cities or counties. Federal policy called the tune. Community mental health centers sprang up around the country. State departments of mental health continued to operate large state hospitals, which backed up the community mental health centers. Also, federal money stimulated the development of ambulatory care in the state hospitals. In a sense, there was a split in the public system between federally funded centers and state funded hospitals. To some extent, this split accounted for the failure of community mental health centers to fulfill a role in caring for people with chronic and persistent mental illness who were discharged from the state hospitals.

The hallmark of the community support period was the re-emergence of state general fund dollars as a major pillar of funding for an evolving public psychiatry. With the repeal by the Reagan administration of the MHSA in 1982 at the beginning of this period, the number of federally funded community mental health centers peaked. States and local communities did not have the resources to continue construction of community mental health centers. Private nonprofit agencies were strapped by the loss of categorical funding during an economic recession. It took time for Medicaid reimbursement to become established and provide a revenue stream for further development. As the decade unfolded, states pursued Medicaid reimbursement to offset general fund expenses, closed state owned facilities, and contracted with private nonprofit agencies for services to their target population. Medicaid benefit structure and reimbursement policies shaped the public system. Also, the rise of

Medicaid established a federal and state partnership reflected in a process of federal review of state Medicaid plans.

With the failure of health care reform under Clinton in 1993, the mainstreaming period of modern public psychiatry (following the example of Medicaid in the decade before) proceeded in full force. In order to achieve the goal of parity in health care insurance, it was necessary to demonstrate the power to control costs in psychiatry, especially after the excesses of private psychiatric hospitals in the decade before. Managed care, despite its rhetoric about quality, was the vehicle for cost control in mental health care and became conspicuous as the face of this period. Managed care in mental health, though tenuously related to accepted clinical practice, achieved its aims via definition of restrictive benefit packages, discriminatory reimbursement policies, and reallocation of fiscal resources from hospitals to ambulatory care. Under managed care, for management purposes mental health services typically were carved out from general health care because of unique clinical and management issues. Carve-outs, which incurred duplicate and high administrative costs, diverted health care dollars from clinical care. The competition between private and public approaches to providing services required that public services reorganize and demonstrate more efficiency. In order to lower costs, alternatives to hospitalization and multiple levels of care emerged in response to the fiscal and financial challenges. The economic recession of 1990-91 accelerated the closure of more state owned hospitals.

> Managed care was the vehicle for cost control in mental health care.

Concurrent with mainstreaming was the appearance of several programs for special categories of patients in needed services. The most conspicuous categories were mentally ill people who were homeless. Another conspicuous group was made up of those embroiled in the criminal justice system. Also, youth becoming too old to qualify for children's long-term, public, institutional services demanded attention. Federal demonstration grants funded the start-up of these categorical programs. Eventually, however, the categorical programs needed to be picked up by state general fund dollars, and they vied for finite, or even diminishing, resources. For example, even as state general fund dollars diminished as a result of the economic recession of 2001, categorical funding for these special populations grew. In the process, the new programs expanded and changed the portfolio of services in the public sector. Also, the change diffused the once-narrow definition of the target population for public psychiatry. Categorical funding and managed care were leading forces shaping public psychiatry in this time.

The 2003 NFC recommended a transformation without new resources from the federal government. The tail end of the economic crisis of 2001, and then the financial crisis of 2008, caused state budget deficits that made state investment in transformation unlikely if not impossible. Essentially, the recommendation for transformation pointed at mainstreaming as the most realistic mechanism for financing the new approaches to care. It would be necessary over time to build into the benefit packages of payers the services needed for special psychiatric populations. The report recommended integration of mental health and primary care. As a corollary, the report deplored the carve-outs of managed care. In these circumstances, the NFC recommendation for integration opened the door for federally qualified health centers—with their favorable, cost-based reimbursement from Medicaid, their eligibility for construction grants, purchase of pharmaceuticals at low cost, and protection from liability—to enter the field of public mental health services. Most community mental health centers explored the possibility of "look-alike" applications to the federal Health Resources and Services Administration and began to collaborate with the community health centers. Better primary care and wellness programs were central tasks for this period. In the case of the state owned mental health center, such as the CMHC, with the arrival of the economic recession of 2008 the only avenue for maintaining services to its population was through encouragement of revenue based service expansion by neighboring, federally qualified health centers.

As the discussion of periods and policies in this chapter have illustrated, diverse variables shaped development of modern public psychiatry and its services. The discussion indicated the undercurrents of politics and economics that were inseparable from (if not preeminent among) the professional, scientific, ideological, and other variables affecting the evolution of public psychiatry over the modern era.

CONCLUSION

This chapter has briefly reviewed the modern history of public psychiatry within the framework of four identifiable periods of development. The framework evolved from a retrospective look at the modern era for the purpose of creating a context for the story of the CMHC. In the press of day-to-day clinical services and the noise of daily administrative and political demands, it is not always easy to know that context. Also, as a function of mainstreaming and management of care, it is sometimes difficult to discern the boundaries of the public sector as people, in the course of an illness, traversed multiple levels of service in both private and public locations.

To the extent possible, the history of CMHC in chapters 4 through 7 is divided into the four periods of modern public psychiatry. It is important to note that the fit is not perfect. For example, the state owned CMHC was protected from some political, social, and economic changes (such as medicating services), or followed a delayed path of evolution. The unique history of the CMHC is a function of its status as a state owned and operated facility with an academic mission. It is not dependent on a revenue stream from entitlements to operate. Also, the CMHC's home state of Connecticut has been slow to embrace Medicaid as a fiscal strategy in order to take advantage of the FMAP. Nevertheless, as the field of public psychiatry evolved in each modern period, it changed the environment in which the CMHC operated and required adaptation by the institution. The policy goals of each period, introduced here, are highlighted in ensuing chapters. Each period also introduced new community services for people with serious mental illness. Those services accrued at the CMHC over the modern era and have created a basis for thinking about future development of the institution.

The State/University Partnership and the Connecticut Mental Health Center

In 1966, the State of Connecticut and Yale University dedicated a brand new institution called the Connecticut Mental Health Center, the embodiment of a partnership. Who exactly were the two partners in this enterprise? What values and cultures did each bring to the partnership? What potential conflicts were inherent in the partnership as a result of the differing values and cultures? How did the CMHC integrate the needs and demands of both partners under one roof as it provided safety-net mental health services to the people of New Haven? How did the institution internally integrate its complex, tripartite missions of services, teaching, and research? The answers to these questions begin to define the character of the CMHC, the history of which this book will trace in the following four chapters.

This chapter provides brief, selective histories and descriptions of the two partners that founded the institution. For the State of Connecticut, the Connecticut Department of Mental Health (DMH) was the agency in charge. For Yale University, it was the Yale School of Medicine through the Department of Psychiatry. The following accounts of the two partners that created the CMHC are selective, chosen with respect to aspects of their history that are relevant to the CMHC itself. No one has written a history of the Yale Department of Psychiatry (YDP). The account here draws on conversations over time with the protagonists of the YDP and the CMHC since the CMHC opened. For the DMH, in addition to conversations with its leadership, the text draws on a chapter from a previous book (Dailey et al., 2007).

THE PARTNERS: THE CONNECTICUT DEPARTMENT OF MENTAL HEALTH AND THE YALE DEPARTMENT OF PSYCHIATRY

To orient the reader, a note on terminology is useful with regard to the Connecticut DMH. This state agency was established in 1954 and, though paying limited attention to addictions, was known as the Department of Mental Health at the time of the opening of the CMHC. In 1973, most addiction services were split off into the Connecticut Alcohol and Addictions Commission (CADAC). In 1996, CADAC was reintegrated with the DMH. The new consolidated agency became the Department of Mental Health and Addiction Services (DMHAS). In the early stages of the history of the CMHC, the text makes reference to the state DMH. In later stages of CMHC development, reference is made to the state DMHAS. The core of the agency, as part of the executive branch of Connecticut's state government and headed by a commissioner who reports directly to the governor, has remained the same since 1954.

The DMHAS is one of the largest state agencies in Connecticut, with more than 4,000 employees. It describes itself as a healthcare service agency and serves over 90,000 people annually. At present, the DMHAS system includes two hospitals and 15 local mental health authorities, of which five are state owned and operated. Through grants, it provides substantial support to 16 private, nonprofit agencies. Its 2009 fiscal year budget was $640 million, made up of state, federal, and other funds.

The YDP is the second largest academic department in the Yale School of Medicine, behind Medicine and above Surgery, and among the largest in the university. The preclinical and clinical education programs include: 80 residents in postgraduate years one through four, 30 postdoctoral fellows, 44 postdoctoral associates, and 24 postgraduate fellows. For the purpose of resident and postdoctoral clinical

> The YDP is the second largest academic department in the Yale School of Medicine.

education, it staffs clinical services at the Yale New Haven Hospital, the West Haven Healthcare Center, and the CMHC. Composing the faculty of the department are 180 full-time and 36 part-time psychiatrists and psychologists. The YDP financial year 2009 operating budget was approximately $100 million. In fiscal year 2009, departmental faculty successfully competed for approximately $70 million in grants for preclinical and clinical research and training fellowships.

Both the DMHAS and the YDP serve adults over the age of 18. The state system serves children under the age of 18 through and a separate agency, the Department of Children and Families. The Yale School of Medicine has a separate, independent Department of Child Psychiatry with the same age limits. These facts deserve mention insofar as they are unusual. In most states and universities, services of academic programs for children and adults are unified. For the most part, therefore, the account of the CMHC in this book restricts its attention to services for adults.

The Connecticut DMHAS and the YDP, the partners in the CMHC, each have primary missions that potentially conflict with the missions of the other. Perhaps the best way to understand the multiple missions of the CMHC is in terms of a Venn diagram (Dailey et al., 2007) (Figure 3-1).

Indeed, often the missions of each partner overlap to generate synergy. The challenge is to achieve the optimal degree of overlap and proper balance. Nevertheless, for the YDP, a commitment to the academic missions of education and research needs to accommodate the state mission to provide services, and vice versa. Conflict can and does occur. Sometimes, academic orthodoxy interferes. For example, in the early history of the CMHC, psychoanalysis—and, later, narrow biological psychiatry—inhibited evolution of the CMHC clinical services by focusing narrowly on particular modalities of treatment and not encouraging a broad spectrum required by people with serious mental illness. The YDP appreciates the task of caring for people with serious mental illnesses and disability but makes little or no commitment of resources to that task. Indeed, the university pursues a policy of not supporting service structures, except for a small, faculty practice that has no relevance for public psychiatry. The DMHAS sustains a primary commitment as to providing services. The commissioner is continuously accountable to the state legislature and the governor for use of the public resources at the CMHC. Often, when resources are short, the large Yale University endowment looms behind discussions of how to reduce costs. Skepticism of academic missions, especially in times of fiscal pressure, is always a background issue.

The potential conflict goes beyond missions and to fundamental values and beliefs. Potential conflict exists between the intellectual "elitism" and the organizational decentralization of academia, an organiza-

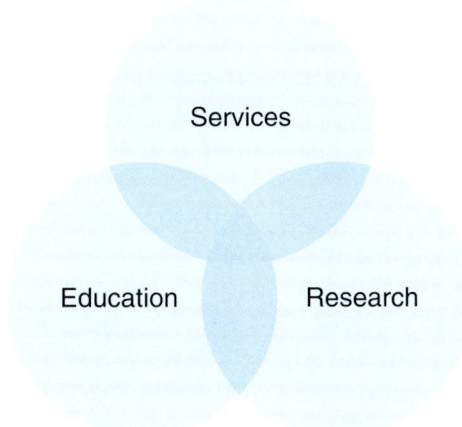

Figure 3-1 Venn diagram of the missions of the CMHC.

tion designed for freedom of expression in teaching and research, and "democratic egalitarianism" of a public, political, and corporate organization of the state, designed to provide public services in a fair way. When either partner loses sight of the potential for synergy between service missions and academic missions, misunderstanding arises and requires active management. The need to monitor and resolve these potential conflicts is a perennial management task.

Indeed, each partner makes essential contributions of resources to the CMHC. This fundamental fact endlessly requires emphasis, especially in times of crisis. Though paid for by the state through a professional services contract, the YDP recruits, prepares, and academically supports professional management for the CMHC. Yale University School of Medicine also commits essential resources to development of research infrastructure and to underwriting of malpractice fees for its faculty and staff (through waiving of overhead costs), and shares indirect research revenues from grants obtained by and located at the CMHC. Also, acquisition of grants brings innovative, supplemental services—carried out according to research protocols—to the patients served at the CMHC. On the other side, the State of Connecticut supports the basic array of services provided to people served at the CMHC by supporting the nursing, social work, and plant maintenance staff, the medical and psychology staff through a professional services contract, and funding for categorical programs.

THE PARTNERSHIP: THE CONNECTICUT MENTAL HEALTH CENTER

The next four chapters provide an account of the Connecticut Mental Health Center from its opening in 1966 to the present. This section in the present chapter introduces the reader to the institution for the purpose of discussing the partnership between the State of Connecticut and the Yale School of Medicine. The CMHC is the institution and the management operation, in which the partnership plays out (Figure 3-2).

The state owns the CMHC and staffs it with nursing, social work, and plant operations. Through a faculty contract, which is essentially a professional services contract, the state contracts with the university to operate the CMHC by providing leadership, management, medical, and professional staff services for the facility. The contract also supports education of psychiatric residents and research by providing for effort on academic tasks by faculty members at the CMHC.

The viability of the CMHC depends largely on the founding document, the Memorandum of Agreement written in 1964 and revised in

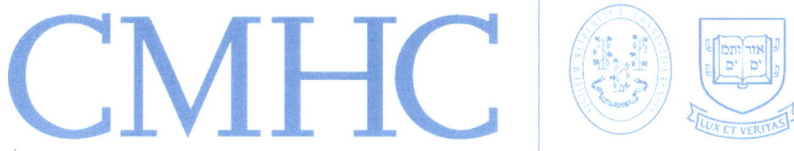

Figure 3-2 The CMHC logo (left) and the insignias of the State of Connecticut and Yale University (right).

1966 at the opening of the CMHC (Figure 3-3). The MOA was revised again in 1978 in order to make budget lines more flexible. The memorandum between the State of Connecticut and Yale University defined the areas of responsibility for each party. The Commissioner of the DMH was responsible for, and had authority over, admitting and treating patients, the use and maintenance of the building, the portion of the budget dependent on general funds of the state, and the performance of state employees assigned to the CMHC. The dean of Yale School of Medicine, through the Chairperson of Psychiatry, was responsible for, and had authority over, the establishment and maintenance of professional standards, the budget through the university (by virtue of the annual faculty and staffing contract or federal funds from grants), and the performance of university employees assigned to the CMHC. The dean and chairperson were also responsible for all research and teaching at the CMHC. According to the MOA, the university nominates candidates for director of the CMHC from its existing faculty or by recruitment of outside candidates. The commissioner appoints the person nominated by the university. The MOA authorizes the director of the CMHC to establish the administrative, supervisory responsibilities and relationships among all the state and university personnel assigned to the institution. The MOA also authorizes the director to provide services, education, and research for the purpose of improving the treatment of mentally ill citizens of Connecticut. The MOA specifies that the director should conduct clinical services and research and education programs. Finally, the MOA describes an annual funding and reporting arrangement for services, training, and research—all seen as mutually dependent. The CMHC budget was broken down into two main parts: the state budget from general fund allocations through DMHAS to the CMHC for building maintenance and state employees; and general fund dollars for the faculty and staff contract that supports leadership, management, medical staff, and psychology staff.

The Connecticut DMHAS and the YDP are the two authorities that continue to define the CMHC up to the present time. It is the state-Yale collaboration that shapes a definition of the multiple missions of the CMHC. It encompasses three missions: clinical services, education, and scholarship. To a lesser extent, the CMHC has over time built community development into its missions, as a product of recognizing responsibilities to the city of New Haven community, where the institution is located. The institution integrates these missions as cohesively as possible in order to achieve balance among them and also to resolve conflict among them. As a function of the basic elements under discussion, the CMHC is a unique, academic community mental health center.

> The CMHC encompasses three missions: clinical services, education, and scholarship.

The appointment and accountability of the director of the CMHC illustrates the relationships in the partnership. The chair of the YDP nominates and the Commissioner of the DMHAS appoints the candidate as director or CEO of the CMHC. The director reports to both the chairperson on academic matters and the commissioner on service delivery. These three individuals are central figures in making the partnership work. They depend on many talented individuals to accomplish their goals. The director of the CMHC is both a full-time, ladder-faculty member (usually a professor) in the YDP and, as head of a major state owned and operated facility, is also a member of the leadership team of the Commissioner of the DMHAS, with respect to facility management. Additionally, the CMHC is a component in a larger system of care for people with serious mental and substance-use disorder in Connecticut. All the leadership of the CMHC, including the chief operating officer, the medical director, and the director of clinical services, are accountable to the two authorities: the Commissioner of the DMHAS for clinical services and state resources, and the dean of the School of Medicine through the Chairman of the YDP. The psychiatrists and psychologists working as clinicians at the CMHC are also faculty in the YDP. By virtue of these joint appointments, the CMHC serves as the principal location of those YDP faculty who concern themselves with academic public psychiatry.

As a final note, it is important to mention that the dichotomies inherent in the partnership and discussion above are little perceived by people seeking services at the CMHC. If anything, the amalgamation of the resources of the CMHC into a unified clinical program of services offers a broad and often innovative array of services for those served at the institution. Even this area of endeavor requires ongoing management of potential conflicts. For example, in order to avoid undesirable interactions among treatments it is necessary to monitor those recipients of care who are registered concomitantly in research protocols and in routine, ambulatory treatment.

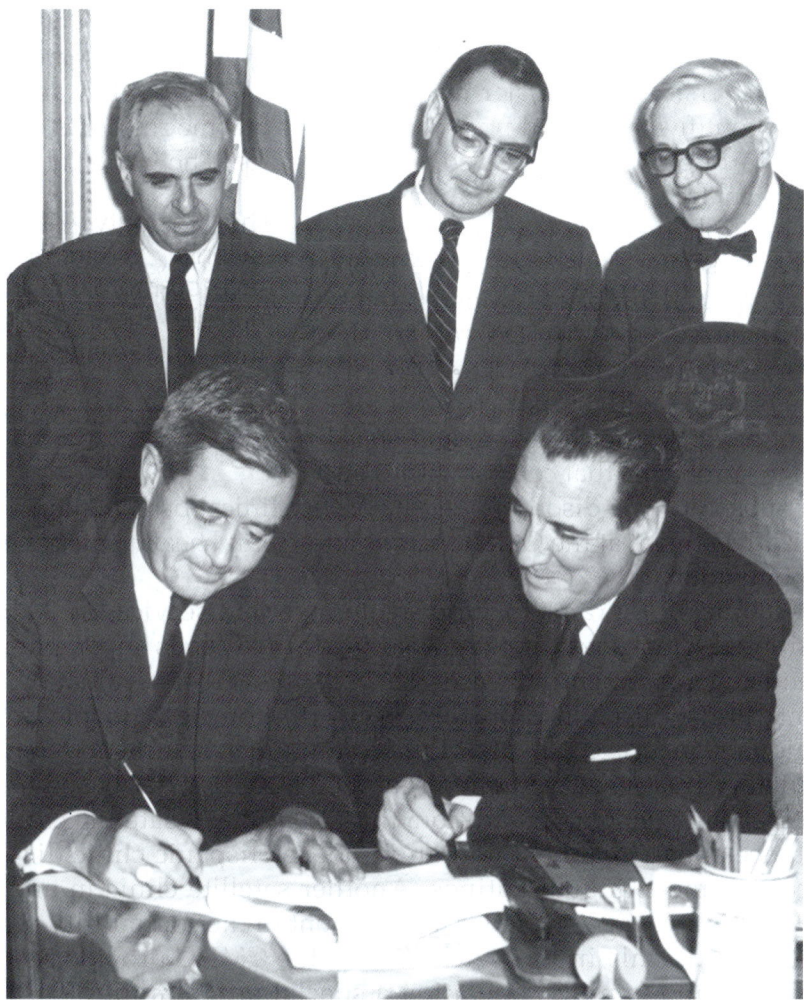

Figure 3-3 The signing of the Memorandum of Agreement between Yale University and the State of Connecticut. Pictured in the foreground are Yale President Kingman Brewster (on left) and Connecticut Governor John N. Dempsey. In the back row (left to right), are Dr. Frederick Redlich, Chairman of the Yale School of Medicine Department of Psychiatry; Dr. John Donnelly, Psychiatrist in Chief of the Hartford Institute of Living; and Dr. Wilfred Bloomberg, Connecticut Commissioner of Mental Health.

THE CMHC AT PRESENT

The CMHC has evolved considerably over the decades. A chronology of major dates and events in the life of the institution is found the next four chapters, which detail that history. The following is a snapshot of the institution at the opening of the second decade of the twenty-first century.

The CMHC is a state owned, academic community mental health center located in a medium-sized urban setting that is dominated by a major university and a major teaching hospital. The CMHC annually serves about five thousand unduplicated, low income residents of New Haven through a variety of clinical programs. The majority of the patients in treatment have co-morbidity from multiple mental disorders, disabilities, co-occurring substance-abuse problems, and legal problems. Most patients are uninsured or have federal entitlements. Many come from large inner-city neighborhoods with typical social problems of poverty, poor housing, and social conflict—problems that coexist with mental or substance-use disorders as part of the clinical presentation at the CMHC. Treatment at the CMHC serves as a mental health safety net for this population.

> The majority of the patients in treatment have co-morbidity from multiple mental disorders, disabilities, co-occurring substance abuse problems, and legal problems.

The clinical programs include: acute inpatient services of 20 beds; transitional, step-down inpatient services of 10 beds in preparation for housing placement; 12 research beds; a walk-in evaluation and urgent care service; an outreach service to homeless people and to individuals in crisis; an assertive community treatment team; an ambulatory treatment program organized into disorder-based teams, and case management. In addition, the CMHC has a satellite clinic for substance-abuse treatment and an in-house Hispanic clinic dispensing care to monolingual Latinos. Another satellite clinic in an adjacent town is a vestige of a federal catchment in the community mental health period. Only in this satellite does the CMHC provide services to children and families, operating a special program for older teenagers and young adults from the city, individuals who are becoming too old to be eligible for state child mental health institutions. Further, the CMHC is a local mental health authority for 17 community-based agencies that provide vocational and psychosocial rehabilitation, residential services, case management, family education, and support services.

The CMHC budget for clinical services from state general fund dollars was approximately $50 million in fiscal year 2009. The total budget for the CMHC in the same year exceeded $80 million. The augmented amount included not only state general fund dollars for special programs but also federally funded and foundation grants obtained by individual faculty. There are about 550 full time and part-time employees, of which about 270 are state employees.

ACADEMIC PROGRAMS AT THE CMHC

Several academic programs integrate into the clinical services. These include law and psychiatry, substance use, gambling, recovery, severe and persistent mental illness including integrated primary care, wellness and health promotion, neurobiology, clinical psychopharmacology, and prevention. A full description and history of these programs is available in the 2007 book, *40 Years of Academic Public Psychiatry*, which documents the history of education in public psychiatry at the CMHC. Psychiatric residents, at all levels of their postdoctoral education, and psychology interns and postdoctoral fellows rotate through the major clinical services. All the academic programs intrinsically have postdoctoral fellows in various stages of research and academic development.

Over time, some clinical services, such as those for substance use, have been more successful than others in accomplishing the goal of academic integration. Some academic programs, such as preclinical neurobiology and, to some extent, clinical neuroscience research, were sufficiently removed from the pressure of services that their academic mission was protected, though their budgets repeatedly experienced pressure. Others, such as the high-volume clinical services of urgent care, crisis intervention, and assertive community treatment, barely allowed enough time for research, though residents did rotate through the services. Generally, certain clinical services have been hard pressed to meet the clinical demand, let alone to follow evaluative or innovative pursuits. This was the result of protecting the academic enterprise—such as the establishment of an urgent care service in 1970 to satisfy the demands of the state—or of a fiscal crisis, or of heightened criticism from the state. Some services, such as substance-use, grew primarily by virtue of research grants or demonstration grants, which protected the research or teaching tasks, and the integration of all missions became a permanent feature of the clinical program. In times of cooperation and good relations with the DMHAS, academic development and integration generally thrived; in times of conflict, such as in the aftermath of crises, academic programs struggled, while at the same time, they provided bridges to the future.

Over time, the policy of the CMHC has been to expect joint appointees—those medical and psychology staff members who are both full-time medical and professional staff members at the CMHC and also full-time ladder faculty in the YDP—to develop independent support from grant applications for teaching, such as T32s, or research, such as RO1s. The critical time for achieving this is in the early years of a full-time academic career. As fiscal pressure persisted over time, the CMHC eventually distilled a policy of supporting roughly 30% effort for academic work for the six years of assistant professorship. It was in this window that joint appointees were expected to achieve not only promotion but also independent support for academic pursuits. By the time someone was promoted to associate professor, the CMHC leadership expected them to support themselves via teaching or research awards or by filling institutional slots in teaching, research, or administration. Also, in 2000 clinician educator positions were developed at Yale Medical School, which facilitated the rise of select joint appointees in positions of clinical administrative responsibility. These individuals were candidates for future institutional leadership in clinical administration at the CMHC, a critical task that is discussed below. By the time joint appointees reach the associate professor level, depending on grant support and the positions they occupy at the CMHC, the effort they devote to academic tasks ranges from 100% (in the case of multiple-grant support) to 10% effort, as everyone in the institution is involved in "bedside" teaching.

THE RELATIONSHIP OF THE YALE DEPARTMENT OF PSYCHIATRY TO THE CONNECTICUT MENTAL HEALTH CENTER

The YDP makes many essential contributions to the CMHC. These contributions are not only a function of the operating principles outlined in the MOA but also of the people who hold key leadership positions in the YDP and the CMHC. Since the first, long-term director of the CMHC enunciated the rule, it has been an internal axiom of the CMHC that you cannot understand the institution without also understanding the people who make it up, and vice versa. The following section considers, over time, the YDP leadership in relation to the CMHC leadership, who were full-time faculty members of the YDP. The discussion highlights the challenges they faced, salient departmental policies, and the consequences of these policies for the CMHC.

The YDP has a long and distinguished history that is a much broader story than that of the CMHC. Arguably, the YDP is one of the most distinguished and largest departments of psychiatry in the United States. The selective account offered here intends to illustrate how the YDP is a key factor in shaping the identity of the CMHC. There is no written history of the YDP on which to draw for this work's purposes. Founding documents of the CMHC (Redlich, 1966) and conversations with the major leaders of the YDP are the sources for much of the next two sections (Jacobs and Griffith, 2007; Jacobs, 1998).

Starting with an overview, it is essential to recognize the contributions of the YDP to the support of teaching and research at the CMHC. Through staff positions paid for by the CMHC, the YDP contributes to the CMHC by providing excellent, centralized administration of resident education programs in basic and advanced public psychiatry, and by providing administrative infrastructure for clinical research. Also, departmental administrative infrastructure for grant administration, again supported in part by budget contributions from the CMHC, facilitates preclinical and clinical research. These supports have grown over the years with centralization of these departmental functions. They are all the more important, too, given contemporary demands for accountability both to funding agencies and to the American Council of Graduate Medical Education. These supports enable the CMHC to sustain itself as an academic community mental health center. Such institutions are a rare breed in contemporary American psychiatry.

At the opening of the CMHC in 1966, Dr. Frederick Redlich was Chairman of the YDP. He was also a founder of the CMHC and its first director for one year. In 1967, he became dean of Yale Medical School. Dr. Redlich was instrumental in creating the modern YDP, and he supported academic program development in neurobiology, psychology, and social sciences. His vision of a broad, diversified, modern YDP served as a guide for the recruitment of a successor.

In 1967, Dr. Gerald Klerman became director of the CMHC. He was a distinguished clinical researcher, who went on to lead American psychiatry in many positions, including as head of the National Institute of Mental Health. As a result of his appointment as director, the positions of chair and director were split. Within a year after his appointment, in response to the turmoil over the opening of the CMHC, which doubled the size of the academic department and occurred in the midst of riots in the New Haven community, the YDP decided to return to the original arrangement, in which the chair was also be the director of the CMHC. Dr. Klerman failed in a bid to become Chairman of the YDP and eventually left the department. In 1968, during a search for a permanent Chairperson, Dr. Theodore Lidz, Acting Chairperson of Psychiatry, became director of the CMHC.

In 1969, Dr. Morton Reiser, a consultation psychiatrist and psychoanalyst interested in a biopsychosocial model for psychiatry, arrived as the new, combined Chairperson of the YDP and director of the CMHC. One year later, he relinquished the director position, in large part because he found the two positions too demanding for one person. His chairmanship was notable for the centralization and development of postgraduate education in the YDP. During his tenure as chairperson, the leading model for psychiatric practice in the YDP was a biopsychosocial model. The department sustained many strong coexisting traditions of inquiry and teaching. Psychodynamic psychotherapy, neurobiology, and social sciences, including epidemiology and services research, thrived. Perhaps the only major school of thought not well represented was behavioral theory and practice. Over time, the development of substance-use programs and interpersonal psychotherapy, among other therapies codified in manuals, gave impetus to these.

> Perhaps the only major school of thought not well represented was behavioral theory and practice.

Stemming from Dr. Redlich's original vision, a departmental biopsychosocial vision provided a broad umbrella and endured for 17 years during Reiser's tenure.

On the CMHC side, Dr. Boris Astrachan was appointed interim director in 1970, replacing Reiser. A year later his position became permanent. Reiser and Astrachan remained essentially coterminous until Reiser stepped down in 1986, and Astrachan in 1987. Astrachan was director of the CMHC for the majority of the community mental health movement and then for the beginning of the period of community services and system development for people with serious mental illness. An expert in resolving conflict within a context of systems theory, his initiative satisfied both the YDP and the DMHAS. As a result, the relationship between the two partners remained stable for many years. During Astrachan's tenure, the CMHC consolidated its position as an institution for teaching psychiatric residents in the YDP. The CMHC annually supported 24 residency positions at various levels, 11 predoctoral and postdoctoral psychology positions, and six graduate nurses. Also, the institution provided a location for both basic and clinical research of the YDP and became the largest and perhaps most important institutional base for it. By the end of Astrachan's first decade, the CMHC had established itself as an essential and stable, fully integrated institutional part of the YDP. It was well on its way to the description above of its status at the beginning of the second decade of the twenty-first century.

Dr. Gary Tischler was appointed Chairman of the YDP in 1986. Since Tischler had started in the department on the federally financed, catchmented Hill West Haven Division of the CMHC, his appointment augured well for departmental attention to public psychiatry. Unfortunately, one year after appointment, he was implicated in an auditing irregularity at the CMHC. As a result, both he and the director of the CMHC resigned in 1987. These departures had enormous implications for both the YDP and the CMHC. The two major leaders in public psychiatry and the YDP were gone in a blink, disrupting planned leadership transitions and leaving leadership uncertainties for two years.

Dr. Benjamin Bunney, who became Interim Chairman of Psychiatry in 1987, was appointed permanently by the dean of Yale Medical School in 1988. He was a neurobiologist and psychiatrist, fundamentally committed to preclinical science. He remained Chair of Psychiatry for 20 years until 2009. His tenure as chairperson was notable for the consolidation and expansion of biomedical research, much of it preclinical, in the YDP. During his tenure, the three major clinical institutions that made up the department—including the CMC, Yale New Haven Hospital, and the West Haven Veterans Medical Center—played a more balanced role in departmental functioning. Also, during this time there was a centralization of research administration and programs, following a centralization of education under Reiser. In 1996, departmental research divisions were added. Investment of limited departmental resources during this period was oriented largely towards preclinical, neurobiological research.

In 1989, Ezra Griffith, a forensic psychiatrist named interim director in 1987, was appointed director of the CMHC. He was director for the last part of the period of community services and system development, and for the early part of mainstreaming. He was faced with the enormous challenge of rebuilding the integrity and identity of the institution and reestablishing the partnership between the DMH and YDP. At this point, the CMHC was supporting the majority of central departmental faculty, who were assigned to department-wide professional and teaching responsibilities. On the one hand, it demonstrated the critical role that the "new" institution for public psychiatry played at this point in time in the YDP. On the other, under the new assumptions of the relationship to the Connecticut DMH, this arrangement was no longer tenable. Educational and special professional roles of central departmental faculty were justified and codified in the annual faculty contract of the CMHC over the next few years. Progressively, the other institutions making up the YDP made appropriate direct or in-kind contributions, realigning institutional relationships under the umbrella of the YDP, and equalizing their roles. In reaction to departmental changes, while keeping pace with the departmental thrust, the CMHC strained to nurture pluralistic models of research and education depending on the needs of patients it served and the demands of a public environment.

Dr. Selby Jacobs was appointed director of the CMHC in 1996. The institutional challenge at the time was to consolidate a strong, generative role for the CMHC, not only in the YDP but also the DMHAS. With respect to the YDP, the CMHC needed to advocate for those academic pursuits that were logically related to the public mission and to demonstrate the academic quality and relevance of those programs. With respect to the DMHAS, the CMHC needed to demonstrate not only its quality and efficiency but also how the academic missions could serve the state through policy initiatives, generation of innovative, grant funded programs, and garnering resources through grants that supplemented the basic, state financed services of the CMHC. Acute care and biological models of practice dominated YDP practice. At the CMHC, psychiatrists had lost touch with responsibility for the disabilities associated with chronic mental illnesses. Attention to rehabilitation was essentially relegated to nonmedical professionals in the community. Jacobs was director during the last part of the period of mainstreaming and the period of transformation.

In 2009, after an interim search period of 18 months, Dr. John Krystal was appointed Chairperson of the YDP. He was a distinguished clinical investigator who translated preclinical discovery into clinical research. Though it is too early to characterize the YDP during his tenure, his first departmental address created a broad umbrella for departmental, academic programs. During the 18-month interim period, Dr. William Sledge was chairperson. In the context of an acute care crisis in American psychiatry, he asserted the needs of Yale New Haven Hospital, the general hospital, where he was concurrently medical director. This initiative directly implicated the clinical services and the community service system of the CMHC. In addition, the YNHH advocated to the DMHAS for relief from the burden of caring for uninsured patients. It forced reconsideration of priorities for both patients in emergency rooms and those leaving the hospital for the public sector, which had been operating under its own community service priorities for the previous 18 years.

In 2009, Dr. Michael Sernyak was appointed director of the CMHC. He was an expert in the treatment of medical problems, specifically metabolic syndrome and diabetes, in people with serious mental illness. A new period of development of public psychiatry was opening up as a result of passage of parity legislation in 2008 and the passage of health care reform in 2010. The combination of these landmark developments stimulated access to mental health and substance-use services by increasing the number of people with nondiscriminatory insurance for mental health and substance-use disorders. At the same time states were facing severe budget problems as a result of the recession of 2008, the worst since the Great Depression.

THE RELATIONSHIP OF THE DMHAS TO THE CONNECTICUT MENTAL HEALTH CENTER

As with the YDP, the contributions of the DMHAS to the CMHC are not only a function of the operating principles outlined in the Memorandum of Agreement, but also of the policies and goals of the DMHAS leadership and administration. Again, consideration is given here to the people who have led the DMHAS over time, their challenges, their solutions, and the consequences for the CMHC and, to a lesser extent, the YDP.

The DMHAS makes essential contributions to the CMHC. It provides a foundation of annual support for the clinical services at the CMHC and also for the academic missions. Through a professional services contract with Yale University the DMHAS underwrites the salaries of medical and psychology faculty at the CMHC, thereby enabling their pursuit of academic missions. The services of the CMHC provide the place for teaching an essential part of psychiatric practice, that of caring for chronically ill and disabled individuals.

Taking a long view over the life of the CMHC, it is worth noting how the organization of the DMHAS evolved considerable over time. The changes had important implications for the relationship of the CMC to the DMHAS. The DMHAS was always a political entity as part of the governor's executive organization. Progressively, it evolved from a professional, essentially medical, organization, led historically by physicians, to a more corporate organization with a CEO, COO, CFO, medical director, legislative and public relations specialists, deputy commissioners, and mid-level managers for special programs such as substance use, housing, or contracting for services under State Administered General Assistance. Connecticut was unique in having a physician as commissioner during much of the modern period. For a period of six years from 1986 to 1992, and subsequent to 2000, clinical psychologists led the department. In 2009, a professional nurse took charge. The combination of nonmedical leadership, a corporate organization, and a diffusion of mission changed the relationship of the CMHC to the DMHAS. It required relationships with multiple people in DMHAS leadership, depending on the task at hand. In the early years of the relationship to the DMHAS, the CMHC leadership largely focused on the commissioner and maybe a deputy. By the end of the modern era, all of the leadership of the CMHC and many of its senior faculty and staff were engaged with the DMHAS central office in strategic planning, policy development, and program planning.

The Connecticut DMHAS has a long and distinguished history (Dailey et al., 2007). The present account picks up at the point shortly after the election of Governor Abraham Ribicoff in 1955. In 1956, Commissioner on Mental Health, Dr. John Blasko, proposed the idea of a "psychiatric diagnostic and treatment center . . . established close to existing medical and scientific research resources." Shortly thereafter, in 1958, Wilfred Bloomberg became commissioner and endorsed the idea, while emphasizing the need for state ownership and control over the institution. It was in 1964, during Dr. Bloomberg's tenure, that agreement was finally reached on a framework for a new institution in New Haven. The agreement was codified in a Memorandum of Agreement.

Ernest Shephard, MD, was appointed Commissioner in 1969. Early in his tenure, the DMH believed that the YDP was too independent in the operation of the CMHC. In short order, however, the commissioner was satisfied by a 1970 clinical reorganization of the CMHC, which essentially created an urgent care service. The CMHC created this new service to meet the demands of the DMH and, at the same time, reassure the YDP that treatment programs used for education were well bounded. The relationship of the CMHC to the DMHAS was stable and cooperative for several subsequent years. While monitoring utilization data to assure state funds were being used to provide services to the people of New Haven, the focus of the DMH in this period was largely on inpatient services at three state owned and operated hospitals. Connecticut made little use of federal dollars to build community mental health centers in this decade. In fact, the Hill West Haven Division at the CMHC was the only example. In 1970, with general fund dollars, the state did open another large community mental health center in Bridgeport, Connecticut's largest city.

In 1976, Dr. Eric Plaut was appointed commissioner. During his term, the DMH pursued a slow and progressive policy to develop community services. The vision of the CMHC, largely set in place in 1970, conformed to the vision of the DMH during this period. The director of the federally funded Hill West Haven Division hosted orientation meetings and provided ongoing consultation to the heads of fledgling private, nonprofit community agencies, some of which would become the future local mental health authorities for Connecticut. Still, the DMH basically maintained a system of state hospitals with clinics attached to the hospital and with little community-based services. At the end of the decade, an additional 100-bed state owned hospital was added to serve the greater Hartford area.

> Dr. Audrey Worrell quickly responded to a pent-up demand in the community for community-based mental health services.

In 1984, Dr. Audrey Worrell became commissioner and quickly responded to a pent up demand in the community for community-based mental health services. Many private, nonprofit community mental health centers got their start in the period following her appointment. To accomplish this change, the DMH had to contend with its own entrenched hospital bureaucracy and also with the general hospitals in Connecticut. The latter brought suit against the DMH for failing to admit as many patients as they deemed necessary, while the DMH was investing in the development of community services. The CMHC supported the DMH in its goal of developing community services, not only by example over its18 years of operation, but also with policy expertise and consultation. In 1982, the state Blue Ribbon Commission on Mental Health reinforced the commissioner's direction. During this period, the DMH opened regional offices to better manage and integrate local services. These offices became an intermediate level of management between the central office and the CMHC. Step-by-step, the DMH began to orient itself toward the care of people with serious and persistent mental illness. As a final note, the growing expertise in forensic psychiatry at the CMHC was instrumental in helping the DMH to build its own programs.

The DMH began to focus on the care of people with serious and persistent mental illness.

Dr. Michael Hogan took over as commissioner in 1986 and continued the policy directions now established in the DMH. A psychologist, he was the first nonmedical Commissioner of Mental Health in Connecticut. He introduced managed service systems, which eventually evolved into local mental health authorities, assertive community treatment programs, and case management. The DMH intensified an almost exclusive focus on people with serious mental illness. This orientation was a challenge to the established academic models in place at the CMHC. In 1987, a crisis in leadership, stemming from audit irregularities, fundamentally shifted the quality of the relationship between the DMH and the CMHC. The crisis caused enormous strain in the partnership between the state and Yale. The economic recession and budget crises in 1989 and 1990 aggravated the situation and became a precedent. Recurrent economic recessions over the next 20 years became challenges for the relationship. During this time, the DMH demanded accountability and implementation of community-based services, while the CMHC struggled to reestablish institutional integrity, meet the demands for service, and regroup its academic programs.

Dr. Albert Solnit, a professor emeritus of Child Psychiatry at Yale University, became commissioner in 1992. During his tenure, the DMH continued to pursue the community-based development of services. It is noteworthy that Solnit had an eight-year term in office, a remarkable fact given the average duration in office of 18 months for state commissioners of mental health. One might have expected the relationship of the DMH with the CMHC to improve. Paradoxically, it did not, for reasons related to long-standing strain between adult and child psychiatry at Yale School of Medicine. Indeed, during this time, the DMHAS made a public demonstration of cultivating a relationship with the University of Connecticut, for the purpose of balance, it was said. In addition, at the expense of the CMHC, which was still catching up after a change in leadership, the DMH elevated the status of the Greater Bridgeport Mental Health Center by heralding its accomplishments. More than once the DMH imposed targeted budget cuts on the professional services faculty contract line item at the CMHC. Following the Robert Wood Johnson model, the DMH implemented local mental health authorities, building on the managed service systems that were intended to create better systems for people with serious mental illness. In 1995 and 1996, under budget pressure and given diminishing census figures, the DMH closed two major state owned hospitals and transferred care of the patients to the community. Also in 1995, the State of Connecticut merged its mental health and substance agencies (the latter having split off in 1972), to form a single agency, the DMHAS. In this process the CMHC played a constructive role as it did earlier in the development of forensic service, insofar as it had integrated mental health and substance-abuse services already in place. Efforts by the DMHAS in 1999 to integrate mental health and substance abuse internally and across the state—despite substantial time and effort—did not move forward as a result of entrenched opposition from substance-abuse agencies. In January 2000, recognizing that Connecticut still had many areas of weakness in its public mental health system, Governor John Rowland called for the establishment of a second Blue Ribbon Commission on Mental Health.

> The CMHC played a constructive role, insofar as it had integrated mental health and substance abuse services already in place.

In May 2000, Dr. Thomas Kirk became commissioner. He was a substance-abuse expert with administrative experience, who remained in office for 10 years, exceeding his predecessor. Following recommendations from the governor's Blue Ribbon Commission and the 1999 Report on Mental Health of the US Surgeon General, the DMHAS embarked upon a process designed to promote use of evidence-based practices, and to more efficiently translate discovery into practice. The DMHAS also actively promoted the use of culturally competent care and set a course for

> DMHAS actively promoted the use of culturally competent care and set a course for development of recovery-based services in the state.

development of recovery-based services in the state. Recovery became another example of fruitful collaboration between the DMHAS and the CMHC, as faculty members of the CMHC provided much of the expertise for this new policy direction. Indeed, this collaboration became a model for building closer relationships between all the academic programs of the CMHC and the DMHAS through faculty/staff positions that split the effort of individual faculty. In 2005, the DMHAS received one of seven national Substance Abuse and Mental Health Services Agency grants to demonstrate a recovery-oriented transformation of the mental health service system, according to the recommendations of the NFC, which reported out its findings in 2003. As an expression of another part of the transformation agenda, the DMHAS also won an award for integrating mental health and substance treatments in co-occurring disorder programs.

Beginning in 2007, the DMHAS began to articulate and publish a strategic vision. The first statement envisioned a value-driven, recovery-oriented system of evidence-based and culturally competent care. In addition, the DMHAS, while striving for organizational and management effectiveness, was developing a quality of care management system and federally funded resources to support its goals. A centerpiece of this policy agenda was the commissioner's intent to have Connecticut, supported by SAMHSA grants, lead the nation on recovery in transforming the mental health service system. With strategic planning now occurring both at the state agency level and at an institutional level at the CMHC, it was possible to forge a strong partnership in pursuit of goals.

In October of 2007, Commissioner Pat Rehmer assumed the leadership of the DMHAS. She was a master's level professional nurse with deep experience in clinical services administration, in both the private and public domains. Formerly deputy commissioner under Kirk, she assumed responsibility for the DMHAS in the midst of the economic recession occasioned by the national financial crash of 2008. Her appointment coincided with new leadership of the YDP and the CMHC. All three new leaders were poised for leadership at the dawn of health care reform in the United States.

THE RELATIONSHIPS ARE RECIPROCAL

It is important to remember that the relationships among the DMHAS, the YDP and the CMHC are reciprocal. The next few paragraphs consider the contributions of the CMHC to the two partners.

The clinical mission of the CMHC, in particular its core mission to serve chronically ill and disabled patients, serves as a reference point for the academic programs at the CMHC. By extension, it does the same for the YDP. In 1966, when the CMHC opened in the context of a psychoanalytically oriented department, many faculty members perceived the CMHC as a threat to their values. Also, faculty members of the YDP at the CMHC, while pursuing the intrinsic intellectual developments in their respective fields, have had to demonstrate over the years the relevance of their endeavors to the clinical mission of the CMHC. These challenges foster a balanced research portfolio and education program. Balance in the YDP might not be achieved in the absence of a facility such as the CMHC. Indeed, this text cites the rise of substance-use programs, law and psychiatry programs, and recovery programs as examples of initiatives that rose in response to challenges in public psychiatric practice. Absent the CMHC, these might not have developed as robustly in the YDP. Ultimately, the clinical mission of the CMHC—while meeting academic standards for teaching and investigation—has become one of the major YDP, medical school, and university commitments to serving the community in which these institutions reside, a fact of considerable advantage to the university in its community relations.

Both the CMHC, as a clinical facility, and the DMHAS face the same basic challenges, including the need to establish evidence-based practice, recovery-oriented care, culturally competent care to reduce disparities in health care outcomes, and development of human and funding resources. In addition, while the state and the university may differ in cultures and in the primacy of particular missions, they share a common interest in meeting the challenges facing the whole field of behavioral health. These include patient safety, quality improvement, patient-centered care, public education, workforce education, advocacy for the field of mental health and substance abuse, and the development of new technology to support these tasks. In all these arenas the CMHC contributes to the mission of the DMHAS.

Through academic initiatives to study new interventions, the CMHC offers innovation in clinical programs. Such innovations supplement clinical resources funded by the state general fund and grants obtained by DMHAS itself. In addition, through its academic programs the CMHC offers policy expertise to supplement the policy experts of the DMHAS. Virtually all the management and academic leaders at the CMHC are actively engaged in work groups for policy development, strategic planning, and particular project implementation or review. Sometimes, when a public crisis arises regarding violent behavior of a seriously ill person in the community, work groups staffed by CMHC faculty members serve as a heat shield for the DMHAS. Furthermore, the DMHAS also has used academic programs at the CMHC as a recruiting strategy to attract qualified professionals to key state positions. The Law and Psychiatry program of the CMHC exemplifies this point. Recruitment for Latino professionals is another example. Recruitment of physicians dually eligible for psychiatry and medicine boards is yet another. The salaries of YDP faculty are so far below those currently paid for state-hired physicians that this strategy also has fiscal advantages in some instances.

ADMINISTRATION IN ACADEMIC PUBLIC PSYCHIATRY

Management of the CMHC offers a case study in the management challenges of academic institutions in public psychiatry. Leadership and management of the CMHC require knowledge and expertise in navigating the two complex bureaucracies of the state and university partners. Within the CMHC there is a need to manage two cultures, embodied in two personnel systems: one deriving from academia for about 280 full- and part-time employees, and the other from a state agency with a civil service system for about 270 state employees. Aside from routine management tasks, such as human resources, budgeting, and facility maintenance, the overriding task for management is to hold the partnership together, while also meeting sometimes competing demands related to services, teaching, and research. Administration is more than the glue of the institution; it is an active process. It demands daily and strategic responding and adapting in a proactive way to the needs and demands of the partners, the services environment, and political and economic developments.

The importance of administration deserves emphasis, as it is the "Cinderella" of the academic enterprise. Academic institutions do not make their reputations on administration. State agencies are accountable for the efficient and effective use of resources for services. The delivery of services intersects with the academic missions. State officials tend to be skeptical about academic missions (Dailey et al., 2007). Academic administration does not have the immediacy and, often times, the urgency of clinical service. Administration suffers from the disdain of academic staff

> Academic institutions do not make their reputations on administration. State agencies are accountable for the efficient and effective use of resources for services.

members, who vigorously pursue their fields of knowledge and discovery and seek to climb the academic ladder. Yet, administration in the CMHC is essential.

Within the CMHC on a daily basis, the concept of an external partnership holds limited significance. Rather, internally, the management challenge is to become part of each superordinate organization that forms the partnership and then pull them together, depending on the circumstances. For example, for the purpose of accreditation by the Joint Commission on Accreditation of Healthcare Organizations, and regulatory review by the Centers for Medicare and Medicaid Services, there is practically no choice as the best strategy for success. The CMHC must integrate the civil service system for state employees and the Yale personnel system for the Yale employees into one office under the supervision of the chief operating officer and a state human resources director. Being part of both parent institutions is an essential aspect of the character of the CMHC. It is also an essential aspect of professional life for those who work there.

Both partners in the productive collaboration between the State of Connecticut and Yale University at the CMHC bring unique histories, cultures, motives, and methods to bear on the facility (Dailey et al., 2007). The task is to pull the missions and cultures together under one roof, founded on the proposition that the three missions of services, education, and investigation, taken together, make the institution stronger. No one can accomplish this task alone. The top leadership of the CMHC is essential in attaining this goal. At the CMHC, a *sine qua non* for success of all the long-term directors, who were physicians, has been a close working collaboration with the CMHC chief operating officer, earlier called the administrator, then the associate director for administration, and their administrative colleagues. This collaboration exceeds other relationships as essential, including academic ones. Over the life of the institution there have been two long-term chief operating officers. The first was Henry Harvey. The most recent over the past 22 years has been Robert Cole, whose skills and commitment to the daily operation and future of the CMHC are notable, though sometimes unnoted.

Budgetary and resource management of the CMHC is unique in quality and is essential, as it is for all institutions. It is this arena in which the COO, who essentially serves as the chief financial officer, plays a crucial role, in collaboration with the director of the CMHC. Both positions require credibility in both the state and the university systems of budgeting, human resources, and facility management. Taking the CMHC budget as an example, it requires accountability to the university for research funds and capital developments in development of laboratory space. In addition, the CMHC purchases educational management from the YDP. The CMHC is accountable to the DMHAS for all three missions of clinical services, education, and research, with regard to the direct state support for the latter missions. It operates human resources within a civil service system, and it operates the facility within plant management structures of the state.

Beyond fiscal and administrative skills, the leadership of the CMHC must actively advocate for the values and budgetary needs of the institution. The CMHC is caught between two cultures and perspectives. State officials consider the CMHC as exceptional, expensive, and expendable, as a consequence of its academic missions. This view prevails despite excellent utilization of services in the community (penetrance) and comparable, if not better, productivity among clinical staff in contrast to its sister state operated facilities. In principle, the university does not finance services. Also, it understands poorly the mission of serving people with serious mental illness. The medical school, as a reflection of its primary commitment to preclinical science and research education, treats clinical psychiatric education and clinical research as a low priority. This state of affairs is not unlike most university medical schools. As is usually the case, the CMHC is exceptional and, if not expendable, not a high priority.

> In principle, the university does not finance services. Also, it understands poorly the mission of serving people with serious mental illness.

The CMHC finds itself in a position where it must demonstrate and advocate for its value. This is not the same as publishing scientific papers, though that is one form of productivity. It involves showing how medical staff members at the CMHC, in part because of comparatively low academic salaries, are a good deal for the state. It involves showing how grants from the federal Department of Housing and Urban Development have augmented residential resources in the community for patients served at the CMHC. It involves reminding the university of the good will generated by the services provided by the CMHC to homeless people on the town green and lowincome people who live in the community. It is a task of understanding what variables are important to the payers and developing data and arguments to demonstrate the value in a pragmatic way. Repeatedly, leadership of the CMHC has pondered if there is a definitive answer to this fundamental challenge of proving its value as an institution. Probably the answer is no. Rather, it remains a task of Sisyphus, carried out endlessly in conversations with state executives, legislators chairing key committees in the Assembly, city officials, and university officials, from the Chairperson of the YDP, through the dean of Yale Medical School, to the president and officers of the university.

The two cultures of the state and the university coexist within the CMHC. Bridging the two cultures and managing the relations between them is an essential task. Each culture has its own values and incentives. The state culture at the level of line staff puts a premium on egalitarian, democratic values and—given a vigorous, unionized work force with multiple bargaining units—concerns itself with job security and formal labor-management relations. The university culture places a value on creativity, initiative, and competition. The university incentives are related to academic productivity, primarily in the form of publishing the results of independent research and obtaining grants to support that goal. The state employees spend 100% effort on clinical services and fulfill 40-hour work schedules (for some unions, 37.5 hours). The Yale employees divide their time among clinical, teaching, and research tasks and work 50- to 60-hour weeks on average, including on-call time. They are not always available for clinical tasks. Grumbling about the differences, and conflict over availability, is common. It is essential to monitor these bicultural work relations and establish integrative strategies to counteract potential conflict. The relationship between the two cultures conflates with, but overshadows, interprofessional relations within the CMHC. In any event, the strategies for managing interprofessional conflict are similar to those for managing the cultural conflict inherent in two distinct work forces.

Integrative strategies for the institution involve the efforts of individuals, creation of a shared organizational culture, mindfulness of the three missions, and shared institutional tasks and procedures. Both DMHAS and YDP employees in key positions at the CMHC play key roles in establishing models for their colleagues in the organization. These include nurse managers, psychiatric attending physicians, and executives. The institution invokes the principle that the CMHC is better than other facilities because it has three missions as an integrative message. The clinical mission of caring for people with severe and persistent mental illness is a major shared commitment of practically every employee at the CMHC and may be the most powerful integrative force of all. Within the bounds of clinical units, the relations between the two cultures and among mental health professions is finessed more easily based on personal relationships and the shared clinical responsibilities. Finally, there are shared tasks, policies, and procedures of the organization for passing regulatory review or solving challenging problems such as disaster readiness, bomb threats, and high-risk clinical problems, such as suicide, which bond the institution together. Holiday celebrations and charitable fund raising endeavors on behalf of the people served at the CMHC also unite the entire workforce.

> The clinical mission of caring for people with severe and persistent mental illness is a major, shared commitment of practically every employee at the CMHC.

The composition of senior management creates a model for the institution, too. Originally, the leadership of the CMHC was made up exclusively of Yale faculty. Over time, the composition of leadership changed in response to budget cuts to the staffing contract for faculty. By 2009, of eight top leadership positions, including the heads of the major mental health professions, three were state employees. They were the nurse executive, the headmnebatk health social worker and the director of Clinical Services. With few exceptions, from an administrative perspective the transition to a new leadership constellation was smooth, aside from the failure in some cases of some individuals to grow into the new level of responsibility. One state employee, the director of Clinical Services, was probably the strongest incumbent in that position in 15 years. She combined an intimate and detailed knowledge of the services at the CMHC (developed from growing up professionally in the institution) with superb interpersonal skills, excellent skills in conceptualizing strategy, service organization, and fiscal management, not to mention outstanding writing skills. There was no falloff between previous university incumbents and this state employee. Another benefit for the CMHC from this change in the leadership constellation was the integration of the university and the state workforces at the highest level, sending a powerful message through the organization.

It is a basic tenet of the CMHC that all the missions are larger and better if integrated together rather than standing alone. For example, the integration of the academic and clinical services missions is important because it makes translation of new discoveries easier. It also contributes to the quality of clinical staff and practice outcomes. Often, academic programs lead in the arena of program innovation at the CMHC, as in the cases of law and psychiatry, substance-abuse services, recovery, and early intervention in psychosis, which have become core programs of the institution. CMHC management advocates for, and protects, the missions when a particular mission, usually one of the academic missions, is targeted for budget cuts. The fact of multiple missions requires that managers communicate continually with policy makers, stakeholders, faculty, and clinical staff about the total picture.

The administrative task in public psychiatry at the CMHC has a unique quality. It involves more than management of the challenges posed by the two partners in the institution. It also requires active involvement in monitoring political and economic developments. This point builds on the discussion of politics and economics in chapter 2 that is the salience of fiscal policies, payers, and reimbursement policies, which form a bridge between policy and practice. Policy is made through politics in the context of economic situations. More than other parts of psychiatry, and perhaps more than any other part of medicine, public psychiatry is inextricably tied up in politics and economics. The account of the four periods of modern public psychiatry at the CMHC in the succeeding text illustrates the role of federal and state political forces on the evolution of the field and the history of the CMHC. It is the administration of an academic public psychiatry institution that primarily engages these issues. If nothing else, the emphasis in

> More than other parts of psychiatry, and perhaps more than any other part of medicine, public psychiatry is inextricably tied up in politics and economics.

this text on politics and economics in management illustrates how managers in public psychiatry at the CMHC think on an organizational and institutional level. In a 1972 paper, the first long-term director of the CMHC referred to this as the politico-economic pragmatics of community mental health. The second long-term director of the CMHC picked up the theme and, in contrast to loftier academic disciplines and in reference to the messy work of legislating, called it "garbage can theory."

Given the essential contributions of effective management over the years, and to sustaining the future of the CMHC as a model of academic public psychiatry, several *desiderata* for success come to mind. Success of the partnership between a state and a university is optimal if the institution and its parent authorities consistently pay attention to providing effective leadership, develop and maintain shared purpose, and employ faculty and staff who are experienced, competent, and respected in both the cultures of the university and the state (Jacobs and Griffith, Chapter 9, 2007).

CONCLUSION

The institution known as the Connecticut Mental Health Center is a partnership between the State of Connecticut and Yale University. It sustains the missions of clinical services, education, research, and to a lesser extent, community development in the neighborhood where it is located. The institution operates within and integrates to the extent possible, the policies and cultures of both parent institutions. Both superordinate partners contribute substantially to the institution. Reciprocally, the CMHC as an institution serves the goals and needs of each partner.

It is not easy to manage the partnership. The evolution of the CMHC over more than four decades is a complex and sometimes problematic story. Yet, it has survived, while many such institutions have not. Though one of many at the outset of modern public psychiatry, it now stands as a practically unique academic community mental health center, serving the needs of lowincome people with mental and addictive illnesses in the New Haven community. The following chapters provide a detailed account of the history and evolution of this institution. Also, foreshadowing a conclusion in the final chapter, the CMHC may serve as an important model for other states and community mental health centers in the future development of public psychiatry.

The Community Mental Health Movement and CMHC, 1966 to 1982

In 1966, the national community mental health movement was gearing up for construction and staffing of community mental health centers across the country. The State of Connecticut and Yale University, under the terms of the Memorandum of Agreement (MOA), were about to open the Connecticut Mental Health Center as a partnership in clinical services, education, and research on the causes, treatment, and care of mental illnesses. Faculty members of the Yale Department of Psychiatry (YDP) were waiting to hear about an application to the National Institute of Mental Health (NIMH) for federal funding to open another community mental health center. This center would be linked to a specifically defined geographic area, called a catchment, in the southwest center of New Haven and the adjoining town of West Haven.

Given the unique, academic character of the CMHC, outlined in the MOA, how did it launch itself into the complex challenges of its tripartite missions? How did it make use of the federal resources offered by the Community Mental Health Centers Act of 1963? In its earliest years, what were the problems it faced in its relation to the state and university, the two partners that formed it? This chapter and the next three tell the story of the CMHC in its formative years and beyond as it traversed the major periods of modern public psychiatry.

ORIGINS OF THE CMHC IN THE POST–WORLD WAR II ERA

The background for the opening of the CMHC in 1966 was the post–World War II era, a time when psychiatrists applying lessons learned about early intervention and prevention during the war formulated a new way of thinking about community mental health. The YDP made seminal contributions to these developments (Jacobs, 1998). Dr. Fritz Redlich, founder of the modern YDP, was appointed chairperson in 1948.

He was a psychoanalyst with broad interests in biological, psychological, and social psychiatry. During the first decade of his tenure, he focused much attention on social psychiatry. He was best known for his scholarly work, completed in collaboration with medical sociologist Dr. August Hollingshead on social class and mental illness. Dr. Theodore Lidz and Dr. Stephen Fleck, both psychoanalysts and leading figures in the early YDP, became interested in the social origins of schizophrenia in families. They conducted research on family communication, which they saw as etiologic in schizophrenic illness and amenable to family therapy. Dr. Fleck was one of the founders of the *International Journal of Social Psychiatry*. Both Dr. Fleck and another psychiatrist, Dr. Jules Coleman, who was also a psychoanalyst interested in novel service systems and therapies, taught in the Yale School of Public Health. In the YDP, the broad range of psychoanalytic theory served well as a framework for social psychiatrists. These highlights illustrate how the YDP was ripe for launching into the brave new world of community psychiatry, which was the new term for the part of psychiatry that fostered the development of community-based services as an alternative to large, overcrowded state hospitals.

The major events and developments leading to the opening of the CMHC, as well as its early years, are summarized in the chronology provided in Table 4-1.

HISTORICAL ROOTS OF THE CMHC

In 1956, shortly after the election of Governor Abraham Ribicoff in Connecticut and the publication by a congressional Joint Commission on Mental Illness and Health on a variety of initiatives to improve the American mental health system, Commissioner John Blasko of the Connecticut Department of Mental Health (DMH) proposed a new state diagnostic and treatment center located close to an existing medical and scientific research institution. About the same time, Dr. Redlich, who coincidentally was President of the Connecticut Mental Health Association (MHA), visited the recently elected governor and asked him what he planned to do for mental health. Governor Ribicoff responded by asking him "What is Yale going to do about mental health?" Redlich returned to New Haven that evening and, with the New York State Psychiatric Institute and the Massachusetts Mental Health Center in mind, drafted a plan that recommended an ad hoc committee of the DMH, the Connecticut MHA, and the YDP to plan for a new institution.

Table 4-1 Chronology at the CMHC of the Period of Community Mental Health, 1963-82

1957	The State of Connecticut and Yale University begin discussions about an institution
1963	Community Mental Health Centers Act
1964	Memorandum of Agreement between Connecticut and Yale University
1966	The Connecticut Mental Health Center opens (Redlich)
1967	CMHC opens the federally funded Hill West Haven Division
1967	New leadership at the CMHC (Klerman)
1967-68	Social upheaval in New Haven
1968	Acting, new leadership at the CMHC (Lidz)
1968	CMHC begins substance abuse services
1969	New chairman of the YDP (Reiser), who is also the new director of the CMHC
1970	New acting director of CMHC (Astrachan), becomes permanent
1973	CMHC begins Latino services
1973	Economic recession
1976	Community mental health movement, second phase, begins
1976	New commissioner of Mental Health (Plaut)
1977	Carter Presidential Commission on Mental Health
1977	CMHC begins Community Support Services Unit for chronic illness
1980	CMHC opens a court clinic, and forensic services coalesce
1981	Repeal of the Mental Health Systems Act of 1980

From the outset, the agendas of academia and the state were different and required extensive discussion and negotiation. The Commissioner of the DMH was worried about Yale commandeering a collaborative institution for the purposes of research and education. The YDP, on the other hand, believed deeply in the role of research and education in creating high standards and advancing knowledge and practice. The YDP was interested in state support of academic missions. The available early documentation (Zeichner, 1970) indicates there was some convergence within a year, by 1958. Dr. Wilfred Bloomberg, who became commissioner

> From the outset, the agendas of academia and the state were different.

that year, supported the idea of a collaborative state and academic center, while also asserting that state control would be important "in collaboration" with the YDP. Over the next six years and through the work of special committees, the concept emerged of a state owned and operated facility in which the leadership, psychiatrists, and psychologists were faculty of the YDP and several joint-appointed nurses were faculty members of the Yale School of Nursing. The MOA between the State of Connecticut and Yale University, finally completed on February 20, 1964, codified the agreement. On the opening of the CMHC in 1966, the two parties wrote a subsequent iteration of the MOA. This document, with minor revisions in 1978 to make budget lines more flexible, still serves as a reference point for definition of the missions of the CMHC, as well as of the respective responsibilities of the two parties in the partnership. An annual faculty/staffing contract between the state DMH and the YDP became the mechanism for paying YDP faculty at the CMHC.

The passage of the Community Mental Health Centers Act by Congress in 1963 (Figure 4-1) and then the Construction Act of 1965 heralded the beginning of a new system of care focused on community-based service and predicated on public health concepts. The new approach was designated the community mental health movement. The passage of these two acts also signaled an active federal role in mental health services. The new movement was the most active federal intervention since President Pierce vetoed the legislation inspired by Dorothea Dix in the mid-nineteenth century. Essentially, the community mental health movement stimulated the expansion of ambulatory services through direct federal funding for construction and staffing of community mental health centers. The new federal legislation created incentives for the Connecticut DMH and the YDP to seek federal grants for saturated

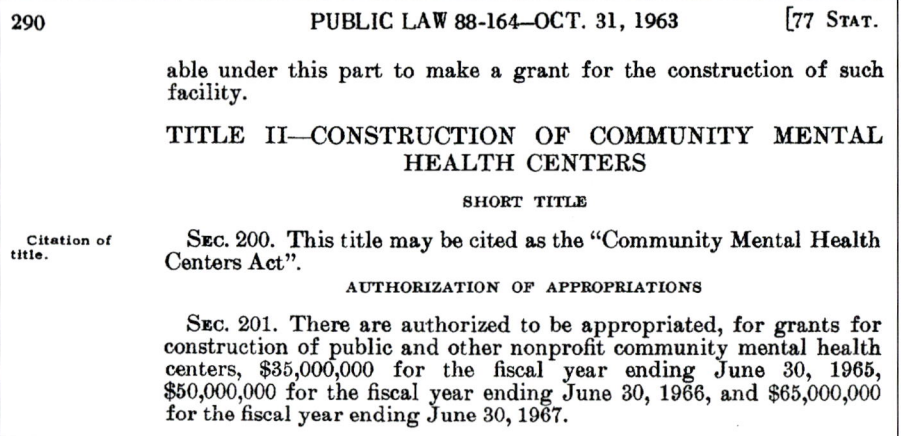

Figure 4-1 Title page of the "Community Mental Health Centers Act" or Title II of Public Law 88-164, Oct. 31, 1063, Construction of Community Mental Health Centers.

clinical services located in specifically designated communities. Federal regulations designated these communities as catchments, which could be no larger than 150,000 people. Regulations required the new community mental health centers to offer five essential services: acute hospital care, emergency services, partial hospital care (day care), outpatient services in clinics, and consultation and education for primary care physicians, courts, clergy, and teachers. These federally funded services offered by the CMHC were dispensed through the Hill West Haven (HWH) Division, which opened as a separate clinical division in 1967, one year after the larger, state funded Connecticut Mental Health Center.

DEDICATION OF THE CONNECTICUT MENTAL HEALTH CENTER, 1966

The CMHC opened its doors in July 1966. The new institution more than doubled the size of the YDP. At the dedication ceremonies on September 30 and October 1, the chairman of Psychiatry, Dr. Redlich, defined the task of the CMHC as serving five major purposes:

(1) to provide exemplary diagnosis, treatment, aftercare, and rehabilitation;
(2) to conduct a broad program of research;
(3) to train mental health personnel, including nonprofessional mental health workers;
(4) to develop models of patient care and training such as day hospitals; and
(5) to participate in the development of comprehensive mental health services for the people residing in the New Haven region.

Dr. Redlich also asserted three areas for special academic contributions by the new institution. They were the epidemiologic study of the catchment area, the evaluation of the effects of mental health efforts, and the development of several mental health professions (Redlich, 1966). He stated that the federally funded HWH Division was a "vivid demonstration of Yale's commitment to the community." Finally, part of the mission of the new institution was "to demonstrate and develop the values and methodology for cooperative efforts between a state government and a major private university" (Redlich, 1966).

By 1967, when the HWH Division opened, the separate and independent federal and state sources of funding essentially created two systems within one building. One was the General Clinical Division, funded with state dollars and governed by the DMH, and the other was the catchment services for the Hill neighborhood and the town of West Haven, funded by federal dollars through NIMH under a federally mandated governing board. Essentially, there was a smaller, and federally funded, center within a larger state funded center, each responding to policies from different origins. Of note, the academic missions of the CMHC fostered teaching and research in the programs of the HWH Division. Reciprocally, over the next 18 years, the services of the HWH Division and federal policies under the 1963 Act were the models that catalyzed the evolution of the services on the General Clinical Division at the CMHC. Also, beginning with the HWH Division and expanding throughout the larger organization, the demands for clinical services at the CMHC progressively shaped the platforms and the agenda for education and, to a lesser extent, research.

THE CMHC IN THE FIRST PHASE OF THE COMMUNITY MENTAL HEALTH ERA, 1966-76

Within a year of the opening of the CMHC in 1966, conflict raged among the faculty of the YDP over the tripartite missions of services, education, and research. Psychoanalysts, representing the leading theoretical discipline at the time, argued with community psychiatrists; academics disputed with community psychiatrists, who were working out on the streets; and psychiatrists, who were political activists, contested with clinical psychiatrists working within the walls of the clinic. In part, the problems were related to a dramatic doubling in size of the academic department. To some degree, the problems emanated from the diversification of academic centers within the expanded department, which was growing not only from the introduction of community psychiatry but also from an ever-larger nucleus of neurobiologists, who were also located in labs at the CMHC. The tension was fueled by large and unexpected service demands at the CMHC. At the beginning of the first year, the CMHC estimated it would log 1,200 contacts annually. Actually, there were 1,600. In the second and third years, there were 2,400. By the end of 1969-70, there were 3,700. To add even greater complexity to these formative years, urban riots in New Haven ignited debate over the role of the university through the YDP in the community.

In 1967, Dr. Redlich was appointed dean of Yale Medical School. Dr. Gerald Klerman, a young, noted clinical researcher, replaced him as director of the CMHC. In the circumstances of departmental conflict, a decision was made at the departmental level to search for a new, combined director of the CMHC and chairman of the YDP. The combined position was designed to better integrate the novel CMHC with the YDP. In 1968, Dr. Theodore Lidz became acting chairperson of the YDP and interim director of the CMHC. In 1969, Dr. Morton Reiser, a psychoanalyst and psychosomatic psychiatrist, was named the new chairman of the YDP and director of the CMHC. This arrangement lasted a year. Then, the new chairperson and director, finding the demands of both positions to be daunting and onerous, appointed Dr. Boris Astrachan as the acting director. The position became permanent the following year. He remained as director for 17 years and was the person whose name is most associated with the early years of the CMHC. Dr. Astrachan was a gifted and committed clinical manager and group therapy expert, who used systems theory as the basis for his organizational thinking. He valued and demonstrated good management. He was instrumental in educating subsequent generations of leadership of the CMHC.

Equally important, the new CMHC leadership was finally successful in 1970 in resolving the intradepartmental conflict. It did so by reorganizing its walk-in, urgent care service at the front door of the institution. The CMHC created an Emergency Brief Treatment Unit and disbanded its day hospital staff to operate it. The institution left unchanged several outpatient treatment teams, which received referrals from this urgent care service and generally engaged in long-term care. Implicit in the reorganization was the concept of crisis intervention and episodic ambulatory care for many individuals, in contrast to the long-term care for those who were referred to the treatment teams. Behind the front door, structures for treatment services remained the same as before, that is to say, organized as teaching programs. Clinicians made referrals to treatment based on vague criteria about suitability for psychotherapy, the dominant treatment of the time. Not only were the criteria implicit, but it was very hard to know at the outset of treatment who was going to need long-term attention. These needs were identified by trial and error over time. The situation was not optimal for serving the needs of people with chronic, disabling illness. It is also important to note that in this time period, the institution defined community psychiatry primarily in terms of its clinical enterprise and not in terms of political or social activism. Social activism was not excluded for those who worked at the CMHC, but it was not considered part of nine-to-five professional responsibility.

> The situation was not optimal for serving the needs of people with chronic, disabling illness.

For more than a decade, the reorganization and decisions just described were the building blocks for development of community psychiatry at the CMHC. The changes resolved the conflict within the academic department about education and research, and proved acceptable to the DMH, which was perennially concerned about access to services for the residents of New Haven. Subsequently, these decisions became part of the teaching lore of the CMHC, serving as a successful example of systems thinking in addressing the complex missions of the institution. Whatever the theory behind it, the clinical reorganization reflected considerable management and political judgment in pulling together multiple competing missions and holding together a complex organization. It is worth putting some emphasis on this discussion, as effective management became an essential part of the success of the institution over time. When leadership and management failed, as it did colossally in 1987, it was a disaster for the institution (see the next chapter).

The HWH Division

In addition to the example of the Emergency and Brief Treatment Unit described above, the federally funded HWH Division, like viral DNA taking over the internal workings of a cell, became the location for implementing and modeling novel clinical programs. This role fulfilled in large part that aspect of the institutional mission to develop innovative services. It was at the HWH Division that socially active and innovative faculty concentrated. In 1966, the original director of the division was social psychiatrist, Dr. Max Pepper. His leadership group included a social worker who was a community organizer and social activist, and a psychologist, who was author of a book about empowering low-income people (Ryan, 1971). Such a leadership group reflected the character of the community mental health movement, including a commitment to social interventions for addressing the presumed, but unproven, environmental causes of mental illness. In 1969, roughly coincident with the arrival of Astrachan as director of the CMHC, Dr. Gary Tischler was appointed director of the HWH Division. The partnership between these two leaders would shape the CMHC over the next 17 years.

The mission of the HWH Division played out within the framework of the community mental health movement and federal policy. The division concentrated services for a geographically defined target population, while providing the five essential services under federal guidelines. The faculty members of the HWH Division were able to show, in a series of studies, that community-based services for a catchment indeed increased access for the target population (Tischler et al., 1972a, 1972b, 1975; Jacobs and Griffith, 2007). Notably, the target population included minority and disadvantaged groups, who historically had been hard to reach. Collaborations with the Yale School of Public Health established a Psychiatric Utilization Review and Evaluation (PURE) project, which became the foundation for mental health services research at the CMHC and in the YDP over the next 20 years. A seminal observation made through the Program Information and Analysis Unit of this program was the 20:80 ratio in service utilization. It was true at the CMHC, and many other similar community mental health centers. In short, investigators documented that approximately 20% of the patients use approximately 80% of the clinical resources. This observation, which would be a recurring theme in the management of resources over the years at the CMHC, led to multiple attempts to better serve this high-utilization and high-risk population.

The HWH Division was the most important link to the community for the CMHC. Federal regulations required community boards in both the Hill neighborhood in New Haven and the town of West Haven, which made up the catchment area. Satellite clinics, both of which routinely made home visits, were located in each community. Community leaders, state legislators, and recipients of care, including their families, engaged with HWH divisional leadership and clinicians. No other part of the CMHC had such a close relationship with the New Haven area. In addition, the HWH Division had to demonstrate annually to NIMH that it was meeting the policies and requirements of the federal grants supporting it. In parallel governing processes, the leadership of the CMHC was accountable to the state DMH regarding the General Clinical Division. The Connecticut statute that established the CMHC created a Community Advisory Board. It was the only board structure for the General Clinical Division. It was advisory by definition and did not intimately engage in monitoring budget, services or other missions. The connections of the HWH Division into the community helped to make the clinical services, and even the academic programs, more responsive to the people served and more sensitive to evolving needs over time.

Multidisciplinary, Clinical Teams

Coincident with the rise of community mental health centers, there was a vast increase in the number of mental health professionals as a product of training grants sponsored by the National Institute of Mental heath (Foley and Sharfstein, 1983). By 1980 the number of psychiatrists had tripled to more than 30,000, psychologists and social workers had more than quadrupled to approximately 59,000 and 89,000 respectively.

This expansion in manpower was designed to correct a shortage of mental health professionals. Many new mental health professionals worked in community mental health centers, and the CMHC was no exception. They filled the ranks of the multidisciplinary clinical teams, which were a novel, basic organizational unit of practice in public psychiatry. The intent was to recreate, in the community, the clinical organization of many psychiatric hospitals.

Conviction about the value of multidisciplinary teams was predicated on the idea that each professional group made essential contributions to the complex clinical tasks of caring for acutely ill and chronically ill people in the community. For example, psychiatric social workers were in charge of assessing and activating social resources and the social environment to make life in the community possible. Psychologists made special clinical assessments, when indicated, evaluated services, and often worked as community organizers. Psychiatrists practiced in the community within these teams, rather than as solo private office clinicians. The CMHC embraced this idea as a fundamental feature of public practice.

During the community mental health period at the CMHC, much time was spent in discussion and clarification of respective professional roles, in light of statutory and professional guidelines. This effort was necessary in order to keep the teams functioning well. But, over time, the multidisciplinary teams also were fraught with obstacles to success. Each professional group believed its role was essential, if not the most important. Even psychiatric aides advocated for social justice on hospital units as a primary goal of care. Roles for each professional group varied over time and required readjustment. For instance, psychiatrists turned from psychotherapeutic to biomedical roles, and nurses from traditional hospital roles to psychotherapy, and then to independent practice. At the CMHC, the division between state and university employees contributed to splits, as the two groups of employees vied for recognition in the organization.

> Multidisciplinary teams were fraught with obstacles to success.

Over the years, interprofessional aspirations and rivalries, which played out primarily on a national level, contributed to the blurring of roles. Nurses and psychologists strived for prescribing roles. Every group aspired to practice psychodynamic psychotherapy, largely a preserve of psychiatrists in the early years of community mental health. When, in the next period of public psychiatry, rehabilitation in the community entered the equation of care, many psychologists and social workers established footholds. Competing models of care—such as narrow psychotherapeutic, biomedical, or rehabilitative paradigms—ignored the full complexity of the clinical task for individuals with serious and persistent mental illness. As cost concerns mounted over the years, some clinical managers questioned the affordability of multidisciplinary teams and defined narrow roles for some, such as psychiatrists, in the name of efficiency. In the face of the forces of fragmentation, effort was required to hold the multidisciplinary teams together.

At the CMHC, the novel multidisciplinary clinical team organization for community-based care worked best on the team level, where the focus was on care of individuals with complex clinical needs. Multidisciplinary professional and in-service education helped to explore and establish team care. Special education programs, notably on the HWH Division, prepared psychiatric aides for more responsible roles on the clinical team, while at the same time these programs responded to community demands for jobs. On an administrative level, CMHC leadership needed to address the goals and frustrations of each professional group in an equitable way (see professional nursing below).

In addition, institutional efforts to support interdisciplinary clinical teams placed a premium on having a working model of care that incorporated all the essential contributions of each professional group in the service of people under care. The theme of team models of care can be traced over the life of the CMHC and is picked up in later chapters. During the community mental health period the prevailing model was rooted in the identity of the institution as a community-based hospital, and informed by public health theories of prevention.

Hospital-Based Services

Following development of urgent care services, the next clinical unit to be organized to respond to the demand for services was the hospital service for the General Clinical Division. All the inpatient services of the CMHC began in 1966 as long-stay, 90-day, 20-bed units. One of them was a clinical research unit—one that remained true to its mission over the next 44 years, though with constriction of resources. Another unit, for the HWH Division, progressively reduced, within a few years, its length of stay from 90 to 30 days. The unit serving the General Clinical Division experienced enormous pressure to expand access to people who lived in the greater New Haven community, excluding the Hill neighborhood and the town of West Haven. Within a few years of opening, the General Clinical Division hospital unit developed a brief hospitalization program that substantially expanded the number of admissions. This program corresponded to the organization of acute care in general hospitals, which were expanding psychiatric inpatient services. The General Clinical Division inpatient unit became part of a general trend to shorten lengths of hospital stay for psychiatric admissions, in part as a function of the 30-day limits of psychiatric hospital insurance benefits. By comparison, other inpatient units operated directly by DMH during this period had much longer lengths of stay and a distinctly custodial atmosphere. Educational and research programs at the CMHC reoriented to the new reality.

THE CMHC IN THE SECOND PHASE OF THE COMMUNITY MENTAL HEALTH MOVEMENT, 1976-81

By 1976, in various parts of the nation 675 community mental health centers were established or under construction. Another 800 were waiting for federal start-up funding. Growing skepticism about a federal role, especially under the Nixon administration, made funding unlikely. In a 1976 amendment to the Community Mental Health Centers Act, the federal government implemented new requirements for community mental health centers. Under federal regulations, enacted in part out of concern that centers were not becoming self-sufficient, seven new services were required in addition to the original five. At the start of the community mental health movement, the original five essential services were:

(1) inpatient;
(2) emergency;
(3) partial hospital (day care);
(4) outpatient; and,
(5) consultation as well as education for primary care physician, courts, clergy, and teachers.

In 1976, the expanded requirements incorporated:

(1) specialized services for children;
(2) also for elderly;
(3) mental health screening;
(4) follow-up and continuity of care;
(5) transitional services out of hospitals for chronically ill individuals;
(6) alcohol- and drug-abuse services; and,
(7) quality assurance.

The amendments also emphasized cross-cultural sensitivity of services and expanded governance by the community. The new federal regulations opened a second phase of the community mental health movement.

Despite these changes, for the CMHC the second phase of the community mental health movement from 1976-81 was a relatively quiet time, certainly in comparison to the start-up period. The compromise between the clinical mission, of central concern to the state, and the academic missions, of central concern to the university, held solid during this brief phase. However, this apparent halcyon time contained the seeds of major change that set a course for more challenges for the institution in the years ahead. Three challenges stand out during the second phase of community mental health movement. One was the implementation of the new federal requirements for community mental health centers. Another was a presidential commission on mental health. The third was the looming need for the HWH Division to become self-sufficient after the statutory limit of 12 years of federal support.

The HWH Division

On the HWH Division all these requirements, including the seven new essential services, were reasonably feasible, eventhough the new federal regulations were a large unfunded mandate. This was true given the broad clinical programs of the YDP and the General Clinical Division of the CMHC. Academic program initiatives within the CMHC, such as the development of a substance-use program and services research, also supported the evolution of services. It was the requirement for transitional services to help move chronically ill people out of the hospital that was the main harbinger of the future. While the HWH Division implemented liaison programs with a large local state hospital, this service for chronically ill people lacked the bold and visionary elements of other centers, such as the assertive community treatment of the Madison model (Stein and Test, 1980). Known as the Madison model, assertive community treatment would eventually spread throughout the field of community mental health. At the CMHC, it was the academic mission that restricted initiatives for people with chronic mental illness. The teaching programs were anchored in traditional hospital and clinic-based services, as well as psychotherapeutic models of care. At the time, patients with chronic mental illness were not considered optimal or even appropriate for teaching and study purposes.

Professional Nursing at the CMHC: Managing Two Cultures and Inter-Professional Relations

Nowhere was the relationship, and often conflict, between the two cultures of the DMH and the YDP at the CMHC more conspicuous than within the profession of psychiatric nursing. When the CMHC opened, nurses were the largest professional group in the institution. Most were state employees. State nurses staffed all the clinical units, filled all the nursing unit management positions and occupied a few other middle level management slots. In addition, 10 nurses who held appointments in the Yale School of Nursing served in unit, divisional, and senior leadership. The relationship between state and Yale nurses, with their separate visions and management systems, was ripe for conflict. Dissatisfaction peaked in 1976, when state nurses were deeply unhappy about insufficient attention they received from Yale nurse executives. Also, all nurses felt unconnected to the Yale leadership of the CMHC. Generally unit-based relations functioned well, where smaller groups got to know and understand each other. After a task force made recommendations to the director, the CMHC leadership appointed a new director of nursing, Ms. Martha Mitchell. Also, a position in the Yale budget line was converted to a position in the state budget line for the purpose of hiring a deputy director of nursing from the state side. This set a course for nursing under the new leadership that lasted for 18 years, in which nursing made essential contributions to the evolution of the institution. For example, nursing leadership played a vital role in advocating for change in the next period of community services and system development for people with chronic illness, though, as the next chapter describes, the leadership as a whole did not respond robustly.

The Carter Commission on Mental Health

Another major challenge and opportunity of this phase of community mental health began in 1977 with the release of the Carter presidential commission on mental health. Just as the 1955 report of the Commission on Mental Illness and Health set a policy direction for the community mental health movement, so did the report of the Carter Commission in the years ahead regarding community services and system development for people with chronic mental illness. The Carter Commission, under the leadership of First Lady Rosalyn Carter, spent one year visiting centers for community mental health across the country. A central preoccupation of the commission was how to render services to the huge numbers of people with chronic mental illness, who were being deinstitutionalized from state hospitals into the community. Most community mental health centers did not effectively address the needs of the population of chronically ill people in the community. The CMHC was no exception. If anything, Connecticut, which did not begin to close its large state hospitals until 15 years later, lagged in deinstitutionalization, but the basic problem was evident within the state and across the country.

The success of the CMHC, a new institution in the YDP, reached a peak at this moment in time. Not only was the CMHC fully integrated into the YDP, with clinical rotations for psychiatric residents at all levels, it also had a vibrant research program. The leadership of the CMHC played prominent roles in the new presidential commission. The CMHC associate director of nursing was a commission member. The director of the HWH Division, who was also a deputy director of the CMHC was appointed deputy executive director of the commission and authored the first draft of the commission report. The director of the CMHC was an active work group member. This level of participation reflected the prominence of the CMHC in community mental health at this time and translated into departmental prominence.

Community Support Services at NIMH and the Mental Health Systems Act

As a reflection of the concern about deinstitutionalization and the presidential commission, the NIMH opened an office of Community Support Services, which would play a key role in disseminating evidence-based community practice over the next 15 years. In 1978 the Carter Commission made recommendations to reorient resources to the problems caused by living with chronic illness in the community. Under prodding from the Carter administration, Congress enacted the Mental Health Systems Act (MHSA) in 1980, one month before the presidential elections. When Ronald Reagan was elected president, his administration quickly rejected a federal role in mental health, echoing President Pierce's rebuff of a national role in extending moral treatment in 1855. In 1981, the Omnibus Budget Reconciliation Act repealed most of the MHSA and replaced direct, categorical federal support for community mental health centers with scaled-back, block grants to states. As part of this change, initiative for implementing mental health policy returned to state departments of mental health. The revocation of the MHSA took some of the steam out of the transition to community services and systems development, at least on a national level. Nevertheless, the ideas embodied in the report of the Carter Commission remained a blueprint for many mental health activists over the next major period in mental health policy development.

At the CMHC, a Community Support Services Division opened in 1977 as a part of ambulatory services to address the needs of deinstitutionalized patients in the community. This unit eventually became the cornerstone of programs on chronic mental illness in the next decade. While this occurred, the central outpatient teaching service relied on a psychotherapy model, one that did not engage people with chronic mental illness or substance-use disorders.

The End of Federal, Categorical Funding for Community Mental Health Centers

The HWH Division was nearing the end of its federal support. Revenues from services were not going to cover the costs of operation, especially given the academic overhead. Within the larger state owned and operated CMHC, revenues returned to the state general fund. CMHC leaders turned in the direction of state ownership to make a transition for the HWH Division. Similar to the case of meeting the 1976 requirements for 12 essential services to qualify for federal support, the larger CMHC subsidized the HWH Division. By 1982, with the start of block grants to states under Reagan, the HWH Division was folded entirely into the larger CMHC.

A few, brief vignettes illustrate some of the cyclical qualities of much of the modern era of public psychiatry. For example, in the circumstances of the economic recession of 1981 and budget deficits, the unique services of the HWH Division that characterized community mental health during the previous 15 years were pared back. Notable in this regard was special attention to the needs of minority populations as a particular target group. It would be about 20 years before attention returned to these critical tasks in the form of a Surgeon General's report on disparities in outcomes for representatives of ethnic and cultural minorities. Special programs in two areas were preserved, but still illustrate cycles. One was a Latino clinic, which continued to grow over the years, as Latinos became the largest minority population in New Haven and demand for service peaked. The other was prevention, which—when the HWH Division closed—was organized into an independent unit, The Consultation Center. Almost 20 years later, the 2003 New Freedom Commission would highlight the need for prevention, and for the promotion of health and wellness.

> A few vignettes illustrate the cyclical qualities of the modern era of public psychiatry.

In contrast to most of the clinical services at the CMHC, the HWH Division and its services were smaller, more nimble, oriented towards federal policy development, engaged with community boards, more oriented to population perspectives, more culturally competent, and generally less constricted by organizational boundaries. The other components of the CMHC, with the exception of the urgent care service, were basically organized as teaching or research units. These distinctions were exactly the reason the leadership over the years had viewed the HWH Division as a model for the development of services within CMHC. The internal reorganization of the CMHC in 1982, when it incorporated the HWH

Division, inhibited efforts to respond to change in the environment of services dictated by federal and, then, state policies. The CMHC lost a division that for 15 years had provided a vision of community mental health, and had been a key agent of change.

The DMH During the Second Phase of Community Mental Health

In 1978, Dr. Eric Plaut assumed responsibility as commissioner of mental health in Connecticut. The state DMH was still staffed by a substantial bureaucracy of administrators and clinicians employed in large state hospitals. It would be four more years before the next commissioner would usher in rapid change toward community-based services. Still, during this phase, the DMH administration began to foster the development of private, nonprofit community mental health centers in Connecticut. Many of the executive directors of these new centers met with the leadership of the HWH Division to learn about community-based services and their implementation. The leadership of the CMHC and the DMH enjoyed amicable and stable relations.

The solution to the fiscal crisis facing the HWH Division as federal funding wound down established an assumption that the CMHC would remain state owned and operated in contrast to the private nonprofit centers springing up around the state and the country. The state ownership of the CMHC served a critical purpose in the new life of the institution. With block grants starting in 1982, and the reemergence of the Connecticut DMH as the exclusive source of support and policy implementation, the CMHC faced the challenge of realigning its clinical programs and academic missions even more closely with the goals of the state agency.

State ownership and governance had ups and downs over the years. On the whole, however, the status of being part of the Connecticut DMH has served the academic CMHC well, despite perennial conflict over the academic mission. For instance, it spared the CMHC the need to "Medicaid" its services, which many private nonprofit agencies pursued during the next 20 years. This pursuit of Medicaid reimbursement required centers to conform to federally approved state plans. In contrast, the CMHC slowly became a part of the Connecticut state agency for mental health. Certainly, the CMHC budget was subject to phases of the economic cycle when state revenues fell. Still, there was an opportunity to work closely with state mental health leadership and policy makers. Sometimes, these relationships were strained, as during the period after a crisis in leadership in 1987 and subsequent years. Ordinarily, it was possible to establish reciprocally beneficial, respectful, and constructive relations for the purpose of sustaining the academic missions of the CMHC. Over the years, the academic missions became unique among community mental health centers across the United States.

ACADEMIC PROGRAMS POISED FOR THE FUTURE

Of note for future development of the CMHC were the strong academic programs emerging throughout the period of community mental health. A forensic unit coalesced in 1979 after successfully securing state funding for a court consultation clinic. This forensic unit became a cornerstone for a law and psychiatry program that would grow into one of the leading programs at the CMHC—and in the country. In the same vein, substance-abuse services crystallized into a substance-abuse treatment unit that later became a cornerstone for development. Both these programs had strong academic foundations, one in teaching and the other in research, foundations that were building blocks for subsequent service development. In addition, demand in services for monolingual Latinos required continuous expansion of services until eventually it was necessary to open a satellite clinic to handle the load. It would take several more years for categorical state support and academic Latino programs to catch up. Another academic program was a prevention unit that rose from the ashes of the HWH Division and became an independent unit. This unit endured as a leading prevention program within the CMHC and the country. The history and significance of these academic programs is developed in subsequent chapters at the point where they came into their own as mainstream components of the CMHC. During the next decade, these programs would play central roles for not only research based at the CMHC but also within the YDP. A full account of these academic programs is available in *40 Years* (Jacobs and Griffith, 2007).

SERVICE DEVELOPMENT FOR PEOPLE WITH SERIOUS MENTAL ILLNESS DURING THE PERIOD OF COMMUNITY MENTAL HEALTH

This and the subsequent three chapters use hypothetical case examples to illustrate the fundamental service developments that supported the process of deinstitutionalization during the period of public psychiatry under discussion. Deinstitutionalization of chronically ill patients from state mental hospitals is the phenomenon that runs as a current throughout the modern era of public psychiatry. These illustrations focus on service development for people with serious mental illness, which is the most needy and vulnerable group, is central to the mission of public psychiatry.

For example, consider the case of Mike, who presents in 1963 to the emergency room of the university hospital in New Haven, with an acute psychotic episode. (Though hypothetical, Mike's case is based on a composite of real patients.) The norm for this time before community mental health was to admit Mike to the nearest state mental hospital, about 40 miles away from New Haven. He spent the next 18 months in the hospital, a duration of stay typical for that time. Recovering enough to be discharged back to his family's home in the community, his chances of relapse were about 80%. His chances were better than 10 years earlier before the prescription of antipsychotic medicine, when chlorpromazine, the first antipsychotic drug, was only in the earliest stage of development and unavailable in his community. Aside from a small teaching clinic in the university hospital, no ambulatory services were available in the community. Mike was given follow-up appointments in the clinic of the state hospital, but essentially he received no follow up because of the hospital's distance from where he lived. Six months after discharge, becoming acutely ill again and reappearing in the ER, he was readmitted to the hospital 40 miles away. On this occasion, his stay in the hospital lasted five years. In 1970, Mike was discharged from the hospital for continuous care in a community-based clinic provided by a new, local community mental health center.

> No ambulatory services were available in the community.

Here is another hypothetical example for the purpose of comparison. Mary fell ill for the first time in 1973, while living in the catchment of the federally funded community mental health center. She presented to the same general hospital emergency room. Mary, in contrast to Mike, was admitted to a hospital service three miles from her home in New Haven. Her length of stay was seven weeks, not months, as a result of the hospital staff engaging her family and social network in construction of family supports for her outside the hospital. She was discharged to a clinic in her neighborhood and followed up by a team of clinicians from the same mental health center that admitted her. She remained at high risk of relapse. Still, the prescription of antipsychotic drugs and supportive therapy of her clinician, including home visits to deliver medicines and evaluate her living arrangements, mitigated the risk. When she became acutely psychotic again, her clinician tried to manage the illness outside the hospital with urgent care, augmented doses of medicine, and intense clinical home visits and social supports. Failing that, she was readmitted to her local mental health center for two weeks. Again, she was discharged into follow-up care in her community. Though Mary's treatment continued over time, this account closes at this point, having illustrated the essential elements of service introduced by the community mental health movement. The example of Mary illustrates not only improved access to care but also improved continuity of care.

Table 4-2 below summarizes the service and benefit innovations of the community mental health period, by contrast with the post-war period in

Table 4-2 Service Type or Benefit by Period of Modern Public Psychiatry		
Service Type or Benefit	**Post–WW II**	**CMH**
Asylum, chronic hospitalization	X	
Acute inpatient hospitalization		X
Nursing home, long-term care		X
Partial hospitalization, intensive outpatient		
Routine outpatient, ambulatory care		X
Emergency room	X	X
Urgent care		X
Crisis intervention		X
Neighborhood clinics		X
Prevention, early intervention		X
Assertive community treatment		
Co-occurring services		
Vocational rehabilitation		
Psychosocial rehabilitation	X	
Case management, community support programs		
Residential services		
System development, local mental health authorities		
Outreach to homeless		
Recovery, quality of life goals		
Peer services		
Integrated primary medical care		
Medicaid Medicare		X
Supplemental Security Income Social Security Disability Insurance		X

Abbreviations: CMH, Community Mental Health; Post–WW II, Post–World War II.

public psychiatry. The system improvements needed to further improve Mary's choices and her chances of recovery would become the goal of the next major period of community services and system development in modern public psychiatry. It is important to note, however, that this improvement in services is only true for those people fortunate to live in a catchment area. Most did not, which was a conspicuous fact at the CMHC. Furthermore, many services needed by Mary at the time she fell ill were not yet available at the CMHC. Missing were the community supports provided by supervised residential placements and money management, and rehabilitative interventions to help Mary recover to the fullest extent possible and be as active in her community as possible. Also, one new level of service, long-term care in nursing homes financed by Medicaid, which Mary avoided, is arguably regressive or at least proved to be problematic. Essentially, the availability of nursing home services fostered a process of transinstitutionalization, which did little to improve the care or quality of life of people with serious mental illness.

SUMMARY

As it might be predicted from the narrative in chapter 3 regarding the State of Connecticut and Yale University as partners in the Connecticut Mental Health Center, a theme emerged loud and clear in the institution during this first period of modern public psychiatry. This theme is the conflict between the demand for services and special service configurations and the demand for creating excellent, productive academic programs. While academic programs thrived during the community mental health movement, there was always a latent (and sometimes explicit) demand on the state DMH for more accessible services and a higher volume of services. This conflict would characterize the entire history of the CMHC.

Nevertheless, the partnership served this academic community mental health center well in its early period of development. State and federal grant dollars undoubtedly provided a foundation for leading, productive academic programs. Reciprocally, initiatives by CMHC academic medical and professional staff established program trajectories in substance abuse, forensic services, Latino services, prevention, and services research that would ultimately prove fundamentally important to the institution and the state in meeting future challenges.

Instantly becoming the largest component of the YDP when it opened in 1966, the CMHC grew remarkably over its first 16 years, becoming an integral part of the department. The CMHC had the largest cadre of faculty and, arguably, by 1982 was the most prominent institution in the YDP, overshadowing the Yale Psychiatric Institute (a freestanding psychiatric hospital owned by the university and devoted to long-term hospital treatment), the psychiatry services at Yale New Haven Hospital, and the West Haven Veterans Medical Center, and the Yale University Health Plan for students and employees. Not only was the CMHC successful in the YDP, but it had established itself nationally as a leading academic community mental health center.

The Community Support and System Development Period and CMHC, 1982 to 1993

5

PUBLIC PSYCHIATRY IN 1982

A new agenda for public psychiatry became conspicuous in 1982. The efforts of the previous five years to plan for an improved, community-based system of care for people with serious mental illness seemed in ruins. The new challenge was to develop a spectrum of community-based psychiatric services and systems for people who were discharged from the hospital, often after long stays, and living in the community. In part, this task was a residue of the failures of the community mental health movement to adequately provide for this population. Development of these services focused almost exclusively on a target population of people with chronic mental illness. Slowly but surely, public psychiatry put in place special services and systems for people with serious mental illness in the community, outside of the hospitals and clinics.

Federal categorical funding for community mental health centers, including the Hill West Haven (HWH) Division of the Connecticut Mental Health Center ended in 1982. Block grants to the state Departments of Mental Health (DMH) began as a replacement for the direct federal support to localities over the previous 15 years. Not only a change in financing, it represented, as part of a new federalism under the Reagan administration, a fundamental shift in program initiative going forward from the federal to the state level. Remaining federal policy initiative would now begin to assert itself through demonstration projects, grants for special categories of recipients, and contracts, for which states could apply and compete. These initiatives included elements of system development such as local mental health authorities or targeted services such as residential services for mentally ill people who were homeless. The Community Support Program office of the National Institute of Mental Health (NIMH) originated many of these, particularly in the first half of the new decade. This office was instrumental in focusing development on the needs of people in the community with serious mental illness through demonstration of programs such as assertive community treatment (ACT). An important backdrop for this change in method of funding and policy initiative was the economic recession of 1981-82, which pinched state and private, nonprofit budgets and required efficiency and pruning of programs.

POLICY BATTLES OF THE NEXT 11 YEARS

Policy initiatives on a federal level during the next 11 years would make surprising and substantial gains for people with serious mental illness. The surgeon general's Plan for the Chronically Mentally Ill, published by the federal Department of Health and Human Services in 1980, served as a guide (Goldman, 1999; Grob and Goldman, 2007). Two examples are signature issues for the new decade. One was disability insurance and the other was Medicaid reimbursement for mental health services.

In 1981, the Reagan administration, concerned with the swelling costs of disability insurance under Supplemental Security Income (SSI) and Social Security Disability Insurance (SSDI), began a review process to reduce the rolls of disabled people. Many people with mental health disabilities lost their disability insurance. Psychiatric advocates mobilized to fight back against a prejudicial review process under the Social Security Administration (SSA). The SSA entered into a dialogue with mental health advocates and began making improvements. By 1984, Congress stepped in and enacted the Disability Reform Act, which required the SSA to cease the review process and institute changes in the review process. The net result was reform in the definition of mental health disability. Also, new procedures eliminated discriminatory practices that inhibited disabled people with mental illness from receiving disability insurance. The availability of disability insurance enabled many people to live in the community by virtue of having a regular income. It was one of the building blocks of the new focus on services and system development in the community.

During the next decade, mental health advocates also enjoyed multiple successes in securing Medicaid reimbursement for poor people with mental illnesses. These legislative successes occurred via a legislative mechanism, the Omnibus Budget Reconciliation Acts, in which the mental health legislation was embedded. Most of the newly reimbursed services were essential building blocks of community services for people with serious mental illness. They included special clinical services, case management, and psychosocial rehabilitation. By supporting community-based services for people with serious mental illness, Medicaid reimbursement unequivocally underwrote the development of a community-based system during this period.

> Medicaid reimbursement unequivocally underwrote the development of a community-based system.

Indeed, some might refer to this time as a Medicaid period, or a period of the "medicaidization" of services by states faced with budget problems, instead of a period of exceptional service and system development (Cutler et al., 2003). With the loss of categorical, federal funding for localities, including the failure of many states to pick up the funding, community mental health centers turned to Medicaid to increase their revenue and sustain their clinical operations. While in the previous decade most community mental health centers had been either federally or state funded, now there was rapid development of private nonprofit organizations under the new funding assumptions. Also, states pursued Medicaid reimbursement of services, in part in the circumstances of economic recession and for the purpose of taking advantage of the federal matching dollars for Medicaid expenses. It was an excellent example of how reimbursement policies under a payer, in this case Medicaid, shaped services and practice for public psychiatry. Also, these developments were a leading example of mainstreaming with regard to a particular payer, which generalized with regard to other payers, and characterized the major policy goals of psychiatry for 20 years beyond this decade.

THE CONNECTICUT MENTAL HEALTH CENTER IN 1982

Over the first 16 years as an institution, the Connecticut Mental Health Center (CMHC) had by 1982 succeeded remarkably both as a leader in the field of community mental health and as a core clinical and academic facility of the Yale Department of Psychiatry (YDP). With the end of the community mental health period, the institution faced the challenge of integrating the HWH Division into a single administrative structure for the entire institution. Despite this large organizational task, the year 1982 opened as a time of great confidence and expansiveness in the life of the institution.

Two factors important to mention here are that the State of Connecticut was one of a handful of states that never aggressively pursued Medicaid matching reimbursement, and the state owned and operated the CMHC. Despite the challenge of absorbing the HWH Division, the combination of these factors protected the institution from the fiscal challenges faced by private, nonprofit agencies during this time. This protection extended not only to the maintenance of most clinical services, but also to the academic tasks of teaching and investigation. Indeed, this insulation from rapid fiscal change proved useful, in general, over the long duration of the institution.

For the first 16 years, the HWH Division had been an engine of change within the larger institution. This division, in response to federal policy initiatives and unrelenting demands for expanding access to services, had introduced most of the service innovations during the community mental health movement. Despite its successes, an important agenda remained for the CMHC. Two areas stand out as examples. For instance, the institution still needed to develop special programs, such as ACT for chronically ill patients in the community. A community support program largely devoted to special service within the walls of the clinic for people with chronic illness was taking shape as a unit of the outpatient division. This program reached into the community, but it did not qualify as an ACT program, which would have required a fundamental reorganization of the entire institution.

Also, unfortunately, psychosocial rehabilitation, as a psychiatric subspecialty—which had a long history as an institutional part of state psychiatric hospitals before community mental health—was not built into the clinical services. In 1982, no expertise on psychiatric rehabilitation, as such, existed within the CMHC. As a result, private nonprofit agencies in the community independently developed rehabilitation services, and a gap opened between treatment services at the CMHC and rehabilitation services in the community. The boundary created by this evolution created a fundamental clinical management task for the CMHC in order to fully meet all the needs of people with chronic, disabling illnesses. These two instances signaled some of the problems that lay ahead.

To orient the reader to this period of public psychiatry at the CMHC, Table 5-1 summarizes the major events and developments.

A NEW COMMISSIONER FOR THE DMH

Dr. Audry Worrell was appointed commissioner of mental health in 1981 and held the position until 1986. She was a community psychiatrist from the University of Connecticut Medical School who had a clear agenda to develop community-based services n the state (Dailey et al., 2007). To do so she had to take on the entrenched, hospital based, state mental health bureaucracy. As if the internal struggle were not enough, as state hos-

Table 5-1 Chronology of the CMHC During the Period of Community Services and System Development, 1982-93

1981	Economic recession
1981	New commissioner of Mental Health (Worrell)
1982	Federal categorical funding ends and HWH Division closes
1982	Federal block grants to states begin
1982	The Consultation Center becomes a center for MH prevention
1984	CMHC program on severe and persistent mental illness begins
1984	Joint Commission on Accreditation of Health Organizations accreditation under hospital standards for first time
1984	Medical and professional staff organization at the CMHC
1985	Partial day hospital opens
1986	Emergency crisis services begin
1986	Ribicoff Research Center of DMHAS moves to the CMHC
1987	New commissioner of Mental Health (Hogan)
1987	Interim leadership at YDP (one year) and at CMHC (two years) following crisis
1988	New leadership in the YDP (Bunney)
1989	New leadership at the CMHC (Griffith)
1989	CMHC begins case-management services
1989	CMHC begins mainstreaming of people with serious mental illness into treatment services
1990	CMHC managed-service system begins and becomes a local mental health authority later
1991	New commissioner of Mental Health (Solnit)
1993	CMHC organizes an institution-wide quality assurance program
1993	CMHC dedicates a building addition as a Substance Abuse Center
1993	National debate on health care reform

pital resources diminished to fund community services, the Connecticut Hospital Association (representing general hospitals in the state) brought suit against the DMH for not admitting patients rapidly enough from their emergency rooms. The DMH, through this new, vigorous leadership, began to drive change within the state. The CMHC leadership developed a strong collaboration with the commissioner to help the DMH achieve the new agenda. As it had been doing for about four years, the CMHC continued to consult with and facilitate the development of private, nonprofit community mental health centers in the state. The time was ripe for the CMHC development of community-based services in New Haven in order to demonstrate new service paradigms.

SERVICES FOR PEOPLE WITH CHRONIC MENTAL ILLNESS AT THE CMHC

The CMHC, in 1982, after absorption of the HWH Division, was essentially organized and operated as it had been since 1970. That is to say as a hospital and clinic, with marginalized clinical services for chronically ill persons and few services provided outside the clinic walls. In short, no fundamental reorganization of services had been made for a target population of chronically ill people. The institution launched a strategic-planning process to prepare for the challenge of caring for people with chronic mental illness in the community.

The strategic planning led to two reports: one on the chronic mental patient and another on improving access to services. Both were flawed, if viewed in the context of the new agenda for public psychiatry. The report on access was predicated on a hospital model rather than on community-based services. A hospital model was consistent with movement in the facility toward first-time accreditation under hospital standards of the Joint Commission on Accreditation of Hospitals (see below). While the access report recommended changes to improve access, the improvements were aimed at facilitating entry to the hospital for brief services and rapid transfer to partial hospital and ambulatory services. Similarly, it recommended briefer treatments in ambulatory care. The access report did not include around-the-clock emergency crisis or wrap-around and outreach services in the community for people with serious mental illnesses, as other facilities in the state were exploring. In short, the report on access was overshadowed by a preoccupation with the hospital status of the CMHC, related to an initial Joint Commission on Accreditation of Healthcare Organizations s (JCAHO) site visit in 1984. If anything, the report on access reflected consistency with models of hospital care that were part of the community mental health movement, not the new period of community services development.

A center-wide, strategic task force on chronically ill patients led to slow and progressive expansion of services for chronically ill individuals. Part of the problem with this report was that it differentiated their treatment from mainstream outpatient treatment, which encompassed individual, group, and family psychotherapies augmented by psychotropic drug treatment. The CMHC leadership invited a leading authority on treatment of chronic illness to consult on the CMHC programs in 1984. One of his comments during his visit was prescient. He concluded that the CMHC was not really organized to serve chronically ill patients. Rather, the CMHC was conspicuously organized for teaching and, to a lesser extent, for preclinical and clinical research. This observation was consistent with the arrangements made 14 years earlier, which were unchanged and done with an eye toward the YDP. The table of organization of the CMHC still used the old system diagrams, which established highly bounded divisions under academic program heads, such as neurobiological

> The CMHC was organized for teaching and for preclinical and clinical research.

clinical research, hospital-based clinical teaching, units, and psychotherapy. It was the CMHC nurses who most consistently advocated for integration of people with chronic illness into CMHC clinical services. For example, they repeatedly made observations about the boundaries between CMHC treatment programs and the state hospital. Furthermore, among leadership, the director of nursing most clearly recognized the need for fundamental, clinical reorganization to achieve the goal.

As the CMHC made gradual, piecemeal initiatives to better serve people with chronic mental illness—and as an outgrowth of the strategic planning process—the CMHC pulled together an academic program on chronic mental illness, drawing on resources from within the YDP. Begun in 1984 by recruiting Dr. John Strauss, a national academic leader in the field, this program was among the first of its kind in the country. It made seminal contributions to the understanding of the possibility of recovery (Wexler et al., 2007). Unfortunately, academic timetables and service-demand timetables were not synchronized. The bold, incipient academic program did not solve the immediate demand for basic reorientation and change. It did set the stage for fundamental contributions and change within the institution in the longer term. For example, a series of studies from this program ultimately challenged the institution to achieve an integration of recovery principles and practices into clinical care. While describing trajectories of recovery, academic attention to chronic illness also provided incentive for better understanding of brain plasticity as part of the agenda of neurobiological research, and the study of innovative interventions, such as computer-based cognitive training to improve work performance.

ACADEMIC CONSERVATISM AT THE CMHC

Serving as a brake on development of new services was another expression of academic conservatism, reminiscent of the conflict between YDP teaching programs and the new community mental health services in the two years after the CMHC opened. The new iteration of academic conservatism was different from the earlier version because the resistance was within the CMHC itself. The leaders of the academic programs at the CMHC were powerful voices, both within the CMHC and the YDP. Their commitment to established teaching models held back change in services. Each faculty member held his or her personal view, consistent with the decentralized organization of academia. Two conflicting goals of the institution created tension: a need to develop a community-based system of services, and a need to maintain full integration into a leading academic department, which was a hard-fought achievement of the previous decade. As late as 1985, the leadership of the CMHC was reluctant to confront the power and academic authority of the director of outpatient services who, while deeply committed to patient care and to teaching, knew little about the new paradigms of community-based services and system development. The CMHC had made itself into a first-class, nationally recognized academic community mental health center. Still, it was not nimble enough to adapt to new models of care in the community for people with serious mental illness. The situation posed a fundamental question about whether education at the CMHC should follow the needs and organization of services, or vice versa. In this particular period, academic conservatism largely won, while later on the need to evolve services led the way.

In fairness to the teaching mission, it is important to recognize that there is a structural component to the issue of change. Once an institution allocates budget to postgraduate medical education, it is hard to pull it back quickly. The institution makes a commitment to the residents it is educating and to the YDP, which constructs an overall education program of a certain size that unfolds over four years. These commitments require time to change, not only within the facility but also in the academic department. In the end, though, it comes down to a question about the content of education during a particular ambulatory phase of residency education. From the point of view of a public psychiatrist, it is difficult to see how allocation of time to focused attention on people with serious mental illness can be shortchanged.

ACCREDITATION OF THE CMHC IN 1984 UNDER HOSPITAL STANDARDS

As part of a national movement, led in part by the American Psychiatric Association, to demonstrate and improve quality of care in general hospital psychiatric units and freestanding psychiatric hospitals, many psychiatric institutions across the country began to submit to regulatory review and seek accreditation from the Joint Commission on Accreditation of Healthcare Organizations. Success in accreditation would provide a seal of approval for the young CMHC. Importantly, the CMHC thought of itself as a hospital, albeit in the community with some community-based clinics. As a reflection of this, the leadership of the CMHC went for accreditation by JCAHO in 1984 under hospital, not behavioral, standards. Successful accreditation reinforced a concept of the CMHC as a hospital, as opposed to a facility primarily engaged in community-based services. To prepare for accreditation, physicians and other mental health professionals were organized into a medical and professional staff.

PHYSICIAN LEADERSHIP OF THE CMHC

Dr. Gerald Klerman, the second director of the Connecticut Mental Health Center, coauthored with Dr. Daniel Levinson a seminal paper on physicians in management, entitled "The Clinician-Executive" (Levinson and Klerman, 1967). The content of the paper was consistent with the assumptions of the community mental health movement, when physicians played many developmental and operational leadership roles in community mental health centers. It was also consistent with the terms of the Memorandum of Agreement of 1966 between the State of Connecticut and Yale University about the leadership of the CMHC. Furthermore, the idea of a physician-executive was a function of the academic character of the CMHC, in which both management and academic qualifications were desirable. The director of the CMHC

> The idea of a physician-executive was a function of the academic character of the CMHC.

and the leadership team had to operate within two administrative structures, not only the state agencies responsible for mental health and addiction services but also the university. Given the size of the CMHC, the former required considerable management experience and skills. The latter required a leader with knowledge, if not success, within the academic system. Though there is an academic department of psychology at Yale University as well as a school of nursing, the MOA specified that the director of the CMHC would be a psychiatrist at the associate professor or professorial level. Social work was not an academic department, and the Yale School of Management took no interest in the operation of the CMHC.

For the most part, the requirement of the MOA for physician leadership served the CMHC well over time. At critical points in the life of the institution it cemented an essential role for psychiatrists. For example, as a result of the loss of federal funding, fiscal hardship, and the economic recession of 1981-82, physicians were systematically losing positions of leadership in community mental health centers. This phenomenon was based on the assumption that they were too expensive to employ in non-clinical roles of management and leadership. Nonmedical, professional managers posed legitimate, lower cost alternatives to medical leadership. In many centers, physicians were no longer even included as medical directors. Rather, they were relegated to writing prescriptions without integrated treatment planning oversight even at the patient level. Given the plight of psychiatrists in the period of community services and system development, the identification of the CMHC as a hospital under JCAHO was understandable in part as a reaction.

The attenuation of physician leadership during community services development also led to disjointed care. The economic considerations mentioned above applied to this development as well. Also, while rehabilitation programs grew in the community, psychiatrists, with few exceptions, were reluctant or slow to lead in this domain. In 1984, the American Association of Community Psychiatrists (AACP) organized to address concerns about the marginalization of psychiatrists in community practice. The AACP advocated for patients and the profession from a medical point of view. Thus, while physician leadership was generally advantageous to the CMHC, it also had its limitations. This was true particularly when conflated with academic identity and in circumstances requiring rapid development of new, nonmedical, or at least broadened, medical service paradigms.

PARTIAL HOSPITALIZATION

In 1985, the CMHC opened a freestanding, partial hospitalization program for people with chronic illness. The new program cannibalized resources originally devoted to a small, ambulatory clinic, which was part of the former HWH Division. Previously, the HWH Division had operated such a program on its inpatient unit as an extension of inpatient care in order to transition out of the hospital. The new program responded to interest in the DMH to better serve chronically ill patients in the community. The partial hospital program offered two strategies for doing so. One was to avert hospitalizations for those people with acute illnesses at risk of hospitalization in the community, which brought them to the emergency room or urgent care at the CMHC. The other was to transition people out of the hospital faster in order to shorten hospital length of stay and increase access. Essentially, shortening length of stay by half doubled bed capacity. The partial hospital program became a platform for essential studies. For example, faculty at the CMHC carried out a demonstration project of the feasibility of providing crisis intervention and respite care to seriously ill people, as an alternative to hospitalization (Sledge et al., 1996a, 1996b).

Because of its 30-day length of stay, the partial hospital program at the CMHC was distinct from many day programs in community mental health centers at the time. In this way it was part of a system of clinical care spanning from inpatient to ambulatory care and consistent with the identity of the CMHC, rooted in hospital and clinic treatment. In most community mental health centers, the day hospital programs evolved into long-term day care and rehabilitative programs. In its time, the partial hospital program was a significant new level of care that foreshadowed the need to develop multiple levels of care during the next period of mainstreaming, when payers managed hospital stays down in order to save money. The demonstration of multiple alternative levels of care with respect to simple, traditional inpatient and outpatient was a product of public psychiatry in the period of community services development. Levels of care were adopted by private, behavioral managed care organizations in the next period of mainstreaming and privatization.

EMERGENCY CRISIS SERVICES

The CMHC introduced crisis intervention services in 1986 as another alternative to hospitalization as part of this progressive change. The CMHC imposed its unique perspective once again on this new service. Instead of embracing the concept of 24-hour mobile outreach in the community to head off ER visits and hospitalizations, the CMHC reverted to what it knew. This was a brief hospital treatment service located within the walls of the hospital, including close collaboration with the ER. This perspective was consistent with the crisis intervention practiced and studied on the HWH Division as part of the community mental health movement. However, these views were out of step with what was happening in community services development of the time, which had veered away from biomedical models and was creating alternatives to hospital care and rehabilitation programs in the community. As a footnote, it is worth saying that the CMHC was later vindicated, when the costs and logistical problems associated with mobile crisis outreach during the night led to retrenchment in public psychiatry to the models proving efficient and effective in the private sector. Years later, the CMHC would implement efficient, mobile crisis services with home visits during day and early evening hours, as this model of service became the norm, not only in the public arena but also the private sector, as an alternative to hospitalization under managed behavioral health care.

A NEW COMMISSIONER OF MENTAL HEALTH

In 1987, Dr. Michael Hogan assumed responsibility as commissioner of mental health in Connecticut. He, and colleagues who arrived with him, came from Massachusetts, which was ahead of Connecticut in the development of community-based services. The DMH pressed ahead with the agenda set by his predecessor. The leadership of the DMH was changing. The new commissioner, a psychologist, was the first nonphysician leader of the DMH. Also, system managers from multiple professional backgrounds joined the leadership team. In contrast, the leadership constellation of the CMHC, which was in part a function of the MOA and in part a feature of the institution under the incumbent director, did not adjust to this change. It remained rooted in medical and hospital versus community support models. Essentially, the director of the CMHC maintained a personal, working relationship with the commissioner of the DMH, and the rest of CMHC leadership had little to do with their DMH counterparts.

In 1986, Congress passed the State Mental Health Planning Act, which authorized small grants to states for planning comprehensive services in the community for people with serious mental illness The planning act gave impetus to regionalization of services and development of all the elements of the Madison model of community-based services as aspects of a comprehensive system. The stage was set for rapid system development. Unfortunately, such development at the CMHC was overtaken by the events described below.

A CRISIS IN LEADERSHIP IN THE YDP AND THE CMHC, 1987-89

As a function of the strategic planning, even with its limitations, and the development of new levels of service, the CMHC began to make slow progress in services development for people with serious mental illnesses. If not for a leadership crisis, the institution might have made it successfully through this challenging period of community services and system development in public psychiatry.

In 1987, Dr. Tischler was appointed chairman of the YDP. Given his background in public psychiatry, his perspective from the Carter Presidential Commission, and his close working relationship to the director of the CMHC, the stage was set for progress to resolve the tension between academic commitments at the CMHC and the need for bold service development. Resolution might have evolved smoothly if not for a crisis in leadership in late 1987.

A routine, state fiscal audit of the CMHC that year discovered inappropriate transfers between state and federal accounts. CMHC administration used state general fund dollars to partially pay the salary of a person who worked neither for the CMHC nor for the university. Actually, an assistant administrator had carried out the account transfer. The finding of the auditors hit the front page of the *New Haven Register* on Wednesday, September 16, (Figure 5-1) but the news had broken in the CMHC two days earlier, which became known later as "Black Monday" in the institution. The director of the CMHC was forced to resign, and the two top administrators were fired. In other words, the top leadership and administrative expertise of the institution were wiped out. In addition, the chairperson of the YDP was forced to resign. The administrator of the CMHC, who was fired, had doubled as administrator of the YDP. All were at risk for criminal prosecution stemming from the audit, though nothing further materialized. A period of investigation by the

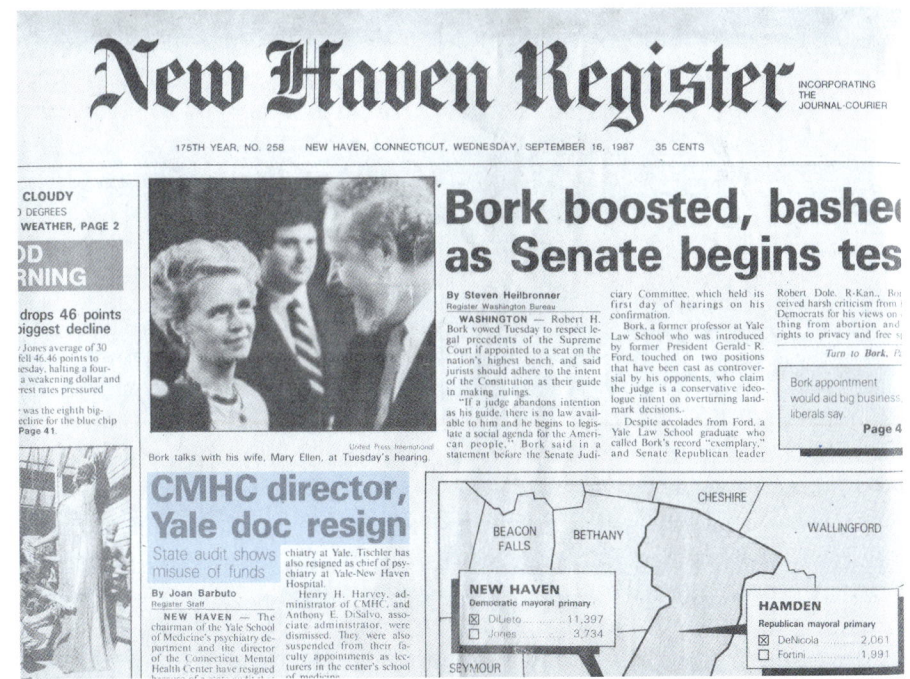

Figure 5-1 Front page of the *New Haven Register* of Wednesday, September 16, 1987, featuring the results of a state audit of the Connecticut Mental Health Center.

state and the university opened. The loss of leadership and the investigation process paralyzed initiative and management of the CMHC.

The audit findings were profoundly embarrassing to both the State of Connecticut and Yale University. On the state side, oversight of financial management at the CMHC was inadequate and not defensible. The sentiment in state government was that the commissioner and DMH had simply turned the state resources over to Yale University without accountability. Officers of the university, on the other side, were forced to question the honesty and competency of psychiatric leadership in the YDP and the CMHC. A relationship of trust and respect that had grown over 21 years tumbled into mutual suspicion, recrimination, and antagonism. The partnership between the State of Connecticut and Yale University came into question.

The circumstances of compromised leadership were ripe for extraneous considerations to drive the agenda. For example, higher order political concerns, which were and are always a consideration in the life of the CMHC, surged in importance in the choice of new leadership of the CMHC. It is important to note, in discussing the politics, that all the candidates for a replacement director of the institution were qualified, excellent, promising individuals. Still, the politics regarding a new parking garage in the local community for the medical center became a decisive consideration in choice of a successor. The vital interests of the state and the needs of public psychiatry did not figure in this political process. Indeed, the interests of the university and medical school had little or nothing to do with the CMHC. It is a cautionary tale of the need for high integrity in leadership and for smooth transitions in leadership for a complex institution, such as the CMHC, to thrive.

THE CRITICAL SITUATION UNFOLDS

The academic character of the CMHC delayed a prompt solution to the need for a permanent, replacement director. The search for a new director of the CMHC was contingent on the search for and installation of a new chairperson for the YDP. Yale Medical School installed a new chairperson about nine months later, after a period of interim leadership and a search process. It was not until more than two years later in November 1989, that a permanent director of the CMHC was chosen. The institution was not rudderless, but it was severely compromised in its capacity to forge a new vision and take new initiatives. It is hard to imagine how far the CMHC had fallen from the heydays of 1979, and the few subsequent years, to arriving at the position in which it found itself—and the challenges it faced—in 1989.

In this time of crisis, mutual suspicions and distrust between the state and Yale surged to the foreground and destroyed the long-standing working relationship that had lasted since its opening in 1966. On the university side, represented by the Yale School of Medicine (YSM), ignorance of public psychiatry, rigidity in the face of crisis, a harshly punitive attitude, and academic arrogance interfered with working out the problem of leadership. On the state side, represented by the DMH, suspicion of the university's motives regarding use of public resources, bureaucratic antagonism to academic missions, and frustration with academic elitism, prevented mutual understanding and agreement. As part of for the process of replacing the director—in which, according the MOA, Yale was supposed to nominate and the state to appoint a new director—a disagreement occurred between the dean of YSM and the commissioner of the DMH. At first, the dean insisted that commissioner could have no influence on the possibility of, or the conditions for, maintaining the incumbent director of the CMHC, which conditions were contingent on the director firing his administrator. The dean then overrode the commissioner's candidate for a successor within the framework of a search process he led. The commissioner was furious about his treatment at the hands of the dean. During the interim period, and even after the new permanent director of the CMHC was chosen, the commissioner essentially decided he would assert his authority in the CMHC, if not attack and punish the university using the only target he had, the CMHC and its leadership. Within the "partnership" between the state and Yale, what should have been mutually respectful and collegial process became antagonistic, divisive, political, and destructive.

During the interim between permanent directors of the CMHC, the leadership was under siege and on the defensive. The DMH regional director became the commissioner's agent on the ground to deal with the CMHC and Yale University. There was closer scrutiny of the budget than ever before. Regional development and implementation of local mental health authorities were placed on a fast track. Services for individuals with chronic illness were fast-tracked, expanded, and mainstreamed.

The relationship of the CMHC to the university was not much better. The chairman of the YDP began to attend leadership meetings at the CMHC, an unprecedented action except for special purposes, in order to keep an eye on the CMHC for the YSM. The best example of the CMHC relationship with the university occurred shortly after the appointment of a permanent director of the CMHC. The university secretary, a former midlevel clinical manger and presumed friend of the CMHC, told the CMHC leadership that she had too much to do to consider the needs of the CMHC. Essentially, the CMHC was left on its own in the local and state political arena. This was a signal development, marking a turning point in the approach used by the CMHC to pursue its political agenda. As a result, the institution needed to start from scratch and build a legislative program to represent its needs within the state and the city. Over time, the CMHC built a network of relationships with state legislators, city politicians, and congressional representatives. It created a need to coordinate CMHC legislative and budgetary pursuits with the goals and framework of the DMHAS, the YDP, and Yale University.

In addition, the YDP needed to put distance between itself and the CMHC. In the process, it reversed a long-term trajectory (if not strategy) of the previous departmental leaders, predicated on a prominent role of the CMHC in departmental financing and management. Indeed, this may have created a conflict of interest in the view of the chairperson, and, in any event, more distance probably was inevitable given the increased oversight of the CMHC expenditures by the DMH. In a sense, the YDP finally resolved a long-standing issue from when the CMHC opened, and doubled the size of the department. The crisis in leadership, the increased scrutiny by the state and, over the next few years, the centralization of research programs (building on earlier centralization of education) cut the CMHC down in size and influence. The new constellation of the department established more equity among the major departmental facilities.

THE CONNECTICUT MENTAL HEALTH CENTER UNDER NEW LEADERSHIP

In 1989, Dr. Ezra Griffith, a forensic and cross-cultural psychiatrist, was appointed director of the CMHC. To say that he had to start over is an exaggeration, but not too far from the truth. The structural aspects of the partnership were in place, but it is hard to imagine the daunting tasks of rebuilding the institution both externally and internally. He was faced with multiple enormous administrative tasks, starting with the most fundamental one of rebuilding a working partnership. In addition, he needed to reestablish the integrity of the institution in all three domains of its three-part mission of services, education, and research. On the state side, under the DMH, it was a time of catch-up to community support programs for people with serious mental illness and with organizational structures to manage a community-based service system. On the university side, the challenge was no less daunting. The leadership of the CMHC needed to build a new relationship with the YDP and regain the confidence of the YMS and university at large.

It is important to appreciate that for a year at the outset, the new director was an associate professor and did not have senior status in the governance of the academic YDP. Though this arrangement was clearly within the terms of the MOA, it was the first time it was true at for the institution. Inevitably, the imbalance in academic rank made the task of leadership more difficult within the CMHC. Many of the academic and clinical program heads with whom the new director needed to deal were already professorial and would vote on the director's promotion to professor, though this situation never materialized into a specific conflict. In addition, the director was deft at managing such inequities and situations. Still, it is likely that it was an important background issue. It is an inequity among professorial members and leaders of the YDP that probably ought not to be repeated. Management of the large, complex CMHC is challenging enough without handicapping the leader.

Part of the aftermath of the crisis in leadership was fragmentation within the CMHC itself. In order to appreciate the task of leadership in this time, it is important to remember the three missions at the CMHC of clinical services, education, and research, not to mention community development. The leadership of the CMHC must expend considerable skill, effort, and judgment on holding these defining missions and the institution together. Other university or state employees at the CMHC ordinarily do not concern themselves with the partnership or with all the missions. Indeed, most staff at the CMHC actively advocate for narrow, more parochial university or state interests. The members of the leadership are the ones who try to judge the allocation of resources and gain buy-in from the staff to advance the whole institution. In addition, the clash of cultures between Yale employees and state employees required active management through informal lunches, holiday parties, and career development for state employees to help them keep pace with Yale-based professionals. Truly, the leadership of the CMHC faced a huge challenge in reestablishing the precrisis equilibrium among missions, staff, and partners.

> The leadership of the CMHC faced a huge challenge in reestablishing the precrisis equilibrium.

The administrative infrastructure of the CMHC also required fundamental reconstruction. A new administrator, who would eventually become chief operating officer, arrived in 1988, during the interim leadership, and faced this challenge. Successful management of the CMHC required credibility in two complex systems of budgeting, human resources, and facility construction and management. Essentially, credibility depended on building personal relationships with scores of individuals in both systems. Also, it required excellent, consistent performance in circumstances in which the demands of each system often conflicted or, even when they converged, needed to be integrated. It was the day-to-day management, typically taken for granted or even under-appreciated by the Yale and state staff of the institution, which helped put the institution back on its feet.

Some clinical and academic programs at the CMHC survived the leadership crisis better than others. Clinical services for the DMH target population of people with serious mental illness, funded by state general fund dollars, were the most impacted. On the other hand, substance-abuse services funded by the Connecticut Alcohol and Drug Abuse Commission were not affected by the crisis. Also, most academic programs funded by federal or foundation grants were essentially untouched. Indeed, many programs pursued aggressive, successful development, unable to wait for administrative stability in order to remain viable. To some extent, independent initiative, discussed further below, contributed to fragmentation in the institution and the need to integrate the missions under an institutional portfolio. It is an example of the complex administrative tasks faced by CMHC leadership in this postcrisis time.

Jumping ahead a few years in time, the twenty-fifth anniversary of the CMHC in 1991 served as an opportunity, and as an early signal, that the institution was beginning to coalesce again under new leadership and was recovering from the crisis that began in 1987. The leadership of the institution used the anniversary as an occasion to bring together figures of historical importance to the CMHC and for the current partners behind the institution to celebrate a distinguished history.

AN ASSERTIVE AGENDA OF THE DMH

The DMH had a head of steam and a full agenda regarding the CMHC. The initiative in service and system development swung strongly to the state DMH. The agent of the state agenda was a regional director of services, who was between the commissioner and the director of the CMHC, a conspicuously diminished relationship. In 1988, during the interim period of leadership, and in response to the demands of the DMH, the CMHC began to develop case-management services, an essential help to people with chronic mental illness living in the community and needing several coordinated sources of services. Also, during the interim in permanent leadership, the outpatient clinic of the CMHC, under a new divisional head, began to develop innovative ideas for integrating the care of people with serious mental illness into the mainstream clinical programs of the CMHC.

In these circumstances of multiple initiatives from the DMH, the CMHC leadership tried to stagger and limit implementation of change, in part to slow the pace of change and in part based on the principle of preserving its academic missions. The institutional reaction not only attenuated initiative in clinical services and in system development imposed by the DMH but also overshadowed initiative on the part of the CMHC itself. It would take more time for the CMHC to become stable and confident enough once again to embrace change as a modus operandi. It was a tough corner to turn, but only by anticipating change and actively searching for opportunities to translate clinical science into practice could the institution hope to regain initiative in service development and make independent and innovative contributions to the DMH.

A MANAGED SERVICE SYSTEM

In early 1990, the CMHC quickly pulled together a managed-service system for the New Haven metropolitan area. This was about three years after the previous director had initiated a work group to make progress in this task, stemming from the federal Mental Health Planning Act of 1986. It is an example of how progress stalled during the difficult transition period after the crisis in leadership. During the transition to new, permanent leadership, representatives of the community were very unhappy with delays in implementation. Newly formed catchment-area councils, designed to formally represent the community, were a major vehicle for expression of dissatisfaction over the delay. With the creation of the managed-service system, which was the precursor of the local mental health authority in New Haven known as the Community Services Network, there was an opportunity to better integrate clinical treatment at the CMHC with rehabilitation and support services in the community.

As a result of concern about fragmentation in the developing community-based services, much attention in public psychiatry was being paid to system development and integration. The accepted wisdom at the time was that integrated systems improved care for the people served. This conviction endured until both a Robert Wood Johnson (RWJ) study and a joint RWJ and National Institutes of Mental Health study, one of the first mental health services research projects, failed to demonstrate better outcomes for recipients of care. At the CMHC, while waiting for the data, progress was made in system development by the coordination of services under an executive committee of agency heads and, in particular, by the eventual formation of a CMHC clinical team linked to residential services in the community. For many years thereafter it was debated whether to integrate or keep separate all ambulatory services and the managed-service system. Both organizational strategies were tried over the years at the CMHC without dramatic change in the function of either side.

A NEW COMMISSIONER

In 1991, Dr. Albert Solnit was appointed commissioner of mental health and remained in office for 10 years. Relations between the DMH and the CMHC in 1990 were strained by the events described above. The appointment of the new commissioner was a harbinger of continuing difficulty. The new commissioner was a former chairman and professor of child psychiatry at Yale University. In contrast to most medical schools, child psychiatry was a separate department at YMS. The relationship of the new commissioner to adult YDP was distant, if not historically strained, in part as a function of his vigorous, notably successful advocacy for children. The net result for the relationship between the new commissioner and the CMHC was that relations were cordial and diplomatic but far from cooperative or, needless to say, supportive. Key examples of this situation were repeated budget cuts to the CMHC imposed by the DMH during the new commissioner's tenure. Typically, academic programs funded through a faculty/staffing contract were used as the bête noir for budget cuts, a surprising turn of events under a commissioner who was a professor emeritus. Given the alienation of the university from the CMHC during this time, the CMHC had to defend itself through the legislative process in order to preserve its academic mission, in particular and, more generally, its identity as an institution with a three-part mission.

FISCAL PRESSURE, LOSS OF RESOURCES AND AN EVOLVING IDENTITY AT THE CMHC

For the next 10 years, starting with the economic recession of 1990-91, budget crises intermittently occurred for state government. All state funded programs at the CMHC faced budget cuts. In order to protect the academic missions from hostile policy makers and bureaucratic actions from within the DMH, the CMHC leadership campaigned for a budgetary line item for the faculty contract. This move would facilitate independent political advocacy by the CMHC. It was a two-edged sword. At the time, given relations with the DMH, it made sense. Once the faculty contract was a separate line item, it was an irresistible target for higher state budget officials looking for cuts in tight times, especially, by their lights, given the enormous endowment of Yale University.

In addition, the state cost of living adjustments for the faculty contract did not keep pace with the annual university salary increases. The net result, independent of annual budget attacks, was shrinkage in purchasing power of the contract over time. Over the next 10 years, 28 positions were lost from the contract. The greatest damage, in part as a function of internal decisions of where to make cuts, was done to academic nursing programs, clinical management, and leadership. But, all sectors of the CMHC were affected to some degree. Over time, inability to pay adequate numbers of medical staff became the limiting consideration in determining the capacity of clinical programs.

The effects of the repeated fiscal crises on academic nursing and nursing leadership best illustrate what was happening on a professional level. Telescoping a long history, starting in 1990, attrition in Yale nurses by 1996 resulted in reduction to only three such positions from an original twelve. By 2004, all these positions were gone. There are multiple explanations for this change. As long as the CMHC saw itself primarily as a hospital and operated three 20-bed units, the role of nursing in the institution was pre-eminent. Eventually, the CMHC evolved away from its hospital identity to one of a community mental health center primarily involved in ambulatory care. Though nurses played a key role in psychotherapy treatment programs in ambulatory care, they were slow to adopt new roles as the tasks of ambulatory care evolved. This change contributed to a diminished prominence of nursing in the organization. Eventually, social workers eclipsed nurses as the largest professional group of the institution. Also, subsequent to the retirement of a long-term director of nursing and her return to direct patient care in 1994, a series of problems in leadership for nursing crippled this professional group over a period of several years. Finally, cutbacks in the faculty contract, which became unrelenting starting in 1990, led to cuts in the Yale nursing positions. Decisions were made to preserve physician positions in part because no alternative, state-funded physician positions were available.

To give an illustration of the effect of fiscal stringency on clinical services during this time, the loss of positions that could be supported in the faculty contract, as well as cuts in general fund dollars, led to reductions in hospital-based services. Acute inpatient services shrank from 40 acute and 20 research beds to 20 acute, 10 subacute, and 12 research beds, a configuration that endures to the present. The partial hospital program, which opened in 1985 and had a distinguished nine-year history, closed in 1994 in the face of budget cuts and the need to fill vacancies in ambulatory care created by a hiring freeze. The choices reflected a new emphasis on, and the need to protect, community-based services in contrast to hospital-based services at the CMHC. The institution was evolving its identity into a community mental health center, which primarily offered ambulatory treatment services, coordinated with community-based rehabilitation and support services through a local mental health authority.

SOCIAL PROBLEMS: DRUG-GANG WARFARE

In the context of both a national and local cocaine-use epidemic, drug-gang warfare and gun violence in the neighborhood of CMHC and in the surrounding community became a challenging and difficult issue. Metal detectors were installed at the front door of the CMHC after weapons were discovered on a clinical unit. Church leaders, other city leaders, and city and state politicians implored that action be taken on the conspicuous social problems of the time. In particular, the CMHC leadership, in collaboration with the New Haven Board of Education, pursued the idea of an alternative school for public high school dropout youth in New Haven. In 1994, the CMHC implemented an alternative school, staffed in part by faculty members from its prevention programs.

HOMELESSNESS

Homelessness was no less a problem. Though having started years before, homelessness was conspicuous on the streets of New Haven. Deinstitutionalization of chronically ill persons from state psychiatric hospitals, along with scarcity of affordable housing in the community, created a challenge of finding a place to live. It was estimated that about 40% of the homeless population was mentally ill, creating complex clinical challenges for those trying to serve them. As people presented for clinical evaluations, treatment planning had to consider options for a roof over the heads of these patients. Optimally, for people leaving the hospital, a spectrum of step-down levels of living were needed, from supervised group homes to personal apartments supported by occasional visits from a case manager. A number of legislative achievements during this time created a foundation for development of residential resources. These included, the Comprehensive State Mental Health Planning Act of 1986, which launched outreach to homeless as an element in the planning process. Also, the 1987 McKinney Act enabled financing of housing for homeless, and the 1988 Fair Housing Amendment Act barred discrimination in housing for mentally disabled.

Building on this federal legislation, the CMHC integrated into a portfolio of services outreach to homeless mentally ill people and housing resources. The institution developed outreach programs for home-less people in order to connect them to clinical and housing resources, thereby offering an alternative to life on the streets and public greens. This direction culminated with participation by the CMHC in the feder-ally funded demonstration research on outreach to homeless mentally ill people described in chapter 6.

THE CITY OF NEW HAVEN AND COMMUNITY DEVELOPMENT

Community development was always the poor cousin in the family of missions for the CMHC. Nevertheless, the CMHC was a major institu-tion in the City of New Haven. To give some idea of this, the CMHC was among the top 10 employers in the city. At the same time, it was a partnership between the university and the state. The city made no financial contribution. Indeed, at times the city was antagonistic, such as when addressing parking needs of state and Yale employees of the CMHC. Still, it was impossible for the CMHC to ignore the conspicuous problems of the surrounding community. In response, it maintained a mission of community development, especially during the second half of its life as an institution.

The CMHC had its baptism in New Haven affairs with the turmoil of 1967-68 during the War on Poverty. The institution then entered a some-what quiescent time during the remainder of the community mental health movement, when federal money dictated the agenda. Once the crisis in leadership was behind it, the CMHC began to engage the city about the problem of homelessness. Early in the next decade, the problem of youth violence called for community initiatives. By rising to action, the CMHC bridged back to the community initiatives of the HWH Division during the community mental health period. The institution followed this direction in part as a function of its development of reciprocal com-munity relations when it came out from under the umbrella of the uni-versity during the crisis in leadership. In the end and, more importantly, the CMHC initiatives addressed a major problem in the local neighbor-hoods and the broader community. It was a building block in extension of the institution outside of the hospital and its clinic boundaries.

CONSTRUCTION AND OPENING OF A SUBSTANCE-ABUSE CENTER

In 1993, the CMHC opened a $3.3 million building addition to house substance-abuse research programs. Faculty and staff of the Substance Abuse Treatment Unit (SATU) took initiative to obtain a National Institute of Drug Abuse (NIDA) construction grant for this purpose. In response, both the university and the state made contributions. The dedication of the building brought together leading university, state, and city officials, as well as NIDA representatives who had contributed to the budget for construction. It signaled the importance of substance-abuse academic program at the CMHC, which had grown over 20 years into one of the leading academic programs of the institution (see below). The new building at the CMHC also elevated substance-use services into full partnership with mental health services. One manifestation of this would be the development a few years later of one of the first special clinical teams for co-occurring disorders. It also provided an opportunity for the partners in the CMHC to renew their commitments to the institution. If it were necessary to find a date when the troubles of 1987 were finally behind the institution, it was probably at this time. It is true that a distant, if not strained, relationship remained between the DMH and the institution, but relations were at least diplomatic.

QUALITY ASSURANCE FOR THE INSTITUTION

In 1993, the CMHC leadership embarked on a quality assurance initiative that was prescient and had far-reaching ramifications. A team of CMHC clinical managers visited the Xerox Corporation, which then had a reputation as a corporate leader in quality and performance improvement. Following strategies learned there, the CMHC began an annual process of setting goals for performance improvement. This process annually focused institutional attention and scarce resources on the most pressing targets for improvement. It served as an antidote to residual sentiments of defeat after the difficult time the institution had just traversed. Also, it served to combat the fragmentation of institutional life after the crisis in leadership by drawing the whole institution together on mutually agreed upon tasks. Finally, it was an early step in quality management that usefully set the stage for an Institute of Medicine report, entitled "Crossing the Quality Chasm," which appeared in 2001.

A NATIONAL DEBATE ON HEALTH INSURANCE

In 1993, the second year of the Bill Clinton administration, the debate about national health insurance was one of the signature policy landmarks of this time. Though never enacted, the debate demonstrated the biases against, and obstacles to, parity of insurance coverage for psychiatric disorders. It also highlighted questions about how to care for people with serious mental illness. As a result, parity of insurance benefits became one of the leading policy goals for the remainder of the decade. The logic for this policy initiative was simple. If the principal means of financing health care would be health insurance, it was essential that psychiatric disorders not be left behind. The policy agenda, though not ultimately achieved until 2008, intended the mainstreaming of mechanisms of financing psychiatric services and welfare benefits for not only the general population but also for people with serious mental illness. The event marked the transition from special facility and system developments for people with serious mental illness, or "exceptionalism," to mainstreaming (Franka and Glied, 2006). The national debate on health insurance during the Clinton administration signaled the prominence of payers in setting the health care agenda. In the future it would become particularly important to understand benefit packages, utilization management, and other financing strategies to understand the direction of developments in public psychiatry.

EVOLUTION OF ACADEMIC PROGRAMS AT THE CMHC

After the crisis in leadership, rebuilding of CMHC as an institution with clinical, educational, and research missions depended in part on decentralized individual efforts within academic programs. Entrepreneurial initiative is standard operating procedure in the research programs as well as advanced postdoctoral research and clinical education. Indeed, during this time at the CMHC, much maturation and development occurred within forensic, substance use, chronic mental illness, and neurobiology within the institution. They helped to prepare the institution and its staff for a broadening of the target patient population and implementation of the clinical programs they needed during the period of mainstreaming. They preserved and developed essential lines of service, expertise, and investigation that might well have been lost in the almost single-minded clinical focus on chronic illness emanating from the state mental health authority. For each of the academic programs located at the CMHC, there was also a departmental valence. Though the YDP did not establish a centralized research division until 1996, the logic of centralization offered a centrifugal force on research within the institution. Therefore, the CMHC was faced with the challenge of fostering a strong identification with the institution. These academic programs became not only pillars of strength for renewal of the institution, but also served as bridges to the period of mainstreaming in modern public psychiatry. A full account of these programs and their long histories is available in another volume (*40 Years*, 2007). The next few sections provide a brief overview.

SUBSTANCE-USE DISORDERS

The development of substance-use programs at the CMHC originated in 1968 when Dr. Herbert Kleber received his first grant from NIMH. At first organized under the name of the Drug Dependence Unit and funded by direct services money from the institute, a core clinical program was methadone maintenance. Over the years, the Alcohol Treatment Unit was started. Federal money was eventually channeled through state service grants to a state agency named the Connecticut Alcohol and Drug Abuse Commission (CADAC), which had split off from the DMH.

In its second decade, the substance-abuse program took off as the result of very successful faculty development and new service demands in the state. American society was in the throes of a cocaine epidemic, making substance use expertise more salient than ever, even while the main approach to the epidemic was interdiction and criminalization under the Reagan administration. The programs of the CMHC consolidated under the rubric of the SATU. SATU provided a foundation for both service and academic programs. In 1993, a Substance Abuse Center, mentioned above as part of recovery from the leadership crisis, opened at the Connecticut Mental Health Center. The substance-abuse group consolidated a position as one of the leading academic programs in the country, while providing indispensable contribution to CADAC. Within a few years, the substance-abuse faculty and staff members of the CMHC were organized into a department of psychiatry research division under the leadership of Dr. Stephanie O'Malley and colleagues (Jacobs and Griffith, 2007).

FORENSIC PSYCHIATRY

Equally productive over essentially the same time was the development of forensic psychiatry programs, which began to form in the 1973 with an elective seminar under the leadership of Dr. Howard Zonana and colleagues. Mental health law grew significantly over these years in cases such as *Wyatt v. Stickney* in 1971 and *Donaldson v. O'Connor* in 1975. These decisions centered mainly on patient civil rights to liberty and patient rights to treatment in the context of civil commitment in state hospitals. The concept of least restrictive alternative for care also developed in case law and eventually became a byword for planning and justifying levels of care. These preoccupations were echoed strongly in the 1999 Supreme

Court's Olmstead decision on the right of patients in state hospitals to the least restrictive and community-based care. A critical interface between the law and practice was created by the Tarasoff decision of 1976, which addressed the responsibilities of psychiatrists, when faced with a patient, who was a high, imminent risk of danger to others. It became essential to understand the law and the roles in control incumbent on psychiatrists.

Under a new name of Law and Psychiatry, forensic psychiatry gained its first foothold in 1979 as a state funded court clinic that provided psychiatric expert opinion and testimony. Coincident with this beginning was a small fellowship program funded by the DMH. Law and Psychiatry, now one of the largest and most distinguished of its kind (Jacobs and Griffith, 2007), evolved into a comprehensive program, not only of expert testimony but also court diversion clinics, alternatives to incarceration, and transition programs for individuals exiting prison. In addition, it served as a resource both for the CMHC and the DMH on landmark developments in state mental health law. The development of forensic psychiatry occurred in close collaboration with the forensic section of the Connecticut DMH. While the developments above augmented the forensic capacity of the CMHC, they also were instrumental in the development of statewide forensic services under the DMH. The CMHC forensic faculty served as expert consultants. They were also augmented state recruitment effectiveness. It was an excellent example of how the academic CMHC could support a key development in public programs at the DMH while establishing a broader base of its own. The Law and Psychiatry program pointed the way for the CMHC in this regard, a path that would be followed in the future by recovery, gambling, and medical programs.

NEUROBIOLOGY AND BIOMEDICINE

Subsequent to the 1980 introduction of the *Diagnostic and Statistical Manual, III* (DSM III), biomedical psychiatry soared in development. It was important for professional psychiatry to establish itself as an evidence-based specialty that could mainstream into medicine. It was equally important for academic departments to better establish themselves within medical schools. Though biological studies of psychiatric disorders had been well under way for 20 years, the DSM III gave the definitions to fuel development.

Neurobiological, preclinical, and clinical research had always been a cornerstone of academic programs at the CMHC (Jacobs and Griffith, 2007). Developments during this time included new antidepressants, atypical antipsychotic drugs, and mood stabilizers. One of the most innovative of these new treatments, demonstrating strength in bridging from preclinical to clinical science, was clonidine treatment for opiate detoxification. In 1986, capitalizing on the imminent closure of the DMH-operated Ribicoff Research Unit at a state facility, named Norwich Hospital, the CMHC moved to consolidate the two programs. Under Dr. George Heninger and colleagues, the new research program became the Ribicoff Research Facility of the CMHC. In the end, as a result of resignations of University of Connecticut faculty at Norwich Hospital, no resources were transferred to the CMHC, save the name.

One aspect of biomedical psychiatry was a two-edged sword for the CMHC. On the one hand, the new treatments coming out of Ribicoff contributed significantly to the care of people with chronic and disabling illness by introduction of strategies for treating nonresponse to first-line drugs, relapse, and management of troublesome side effects of drugs. The Ribicoff leadership at the CMHC, many of whom strongly identified with the clinical mission of the institution, helped to sustain and rebuild the relationship to YDP. The Ribicoff faculty also brought tangible benefit in the form of a commitment of the medical school and the state to building yet another addition to the CMHC, a development covered chapter 7. On the other hand, while biomedical research brought new treatments, it also compartmentalized medical and social aspects of illness as well as treatment and psychosocial rehabilitation. This development posed challenges for the care of chronically ill individuals. In its narrow preoccupation with diagnosis and its emphasis on pharmacologic treatments, biological psychiatry was not broad enough for the challenge to develop community-based services. In its adoption of a narrow medical model, it was reminiscent of the earlier hospital-based practice in the pubic sector, before the community mental health movement, though, in the new iteration, it played out on both hospital and ambulatory platforms. It failed to connect with rehabilitation as asylum-based practice had done.

EDUCATION AND THE RELATIONSHIP BETWEEN TEACHING AND SERVICES

Much to the credit of the leadership and faculty of the CMHC during the phase of rebuilding the institution, a commitment to educational programs endured steady and stable. The institution sustained teaching programs for psychiatric residents at basic and advanced levels of their education, including advanced training in public psychiatry (Jacobs and Griffith, 2007). Education of predoc and postdoc psychologists continued as well. Though master's level education for nurses was tailing off, nursing rotations for several local nursing schools thrived. Social work students also used the CMHC for clinical placements.

One consequence of the changes in the postcrisis period was an evolution in attitude about the relationship between teaching and services. The services required by patients with serious mental illness, and by evolving concepts of service, became a leading consideration within educational programs at the CMHC. The institution needed to fit within the landscape of new service paradigms for people with serious mental illness envisioned by the DMH. In addition, it needed to strive once again for a leading role in providing clinical services in the public system. Through teaching, the CMHC could make a fundamental contribution to preparation of new generations of mental health professionals, who would work in the public sphere. This is the only appropriate role for an academic community mental health center, and a fundamental justification of its public support.

CONSEQUENCES OF SERVICE DEVELOPMENT FOR CLINICAL PRACTICE AT THE CMHC

While biological psychiatry was retrenching into a narrow model of diagnosis and biomedical treatment that excluded attention to the social and environmental variables, other conflicting forces were at play. Progressively, deinstitutionalization under the Reagan administration combined with the criminalization of substance abuse and bizarre behavior, ratcheted up the numbers of two populations seen at the front door of the CMHC. Over several years, patients involved with the criminal justice system or having substance-use problems were modal and not the exceptions. People no longer presented to the CMHC with a single disorder but rather with co-occurring disorder, while under arrest, or with charges pending, or on court diversion. Treatments for addictions and clinical care for individuals involved in the criminal justice system became major streams of service. These changes, including the social problem of homelessness described above, considerably complicated clinical evaluation and treatment of individuals presenting to the CMHC.

> Treatments for addictions and clinical care for individuals involved in the criminal justice system became major streams of service.

The changes in the patient population challenged established clinical cultures in more than one way. For example, the original and traditional treatment philosophy in substance-use programs differed from mental health in being more confrontational and medically oriented than the psychotherapy-based, ambulatory services at the CMHC. Culture conflict between the two clinical camps occurred in regard to judgments about motivation for seeking care and outreach. The gap that existed between primary assignment to one type of treatment or another was a limbo in accessing services, into which applicants for care often fell. Difficult and time-consuming as the conflict was, it was a useful beginning of a dialogue, which still goes on and which prepared the CMHC for a later development of special clinical programs for people with co-occurring disorders. Another example of clinical culture conflict was the challenge to reevaluate a traditional, psychotherapeutic rule that you needed to be motivated for treatment in order to benefit from it. It became clear from experience, and eventually systematic data to support it, that many patients profited from treatment even when mandated to care.

Debates about these issues were prominent parts of clinical life during this period of public psychiatry. It was not for another several years that the changes in patient population and clinical culture were conspicuous, and when the CMHC began to discuss a noticeable diffusion in the target population. Still, paradoxically, the seeds were sown during this period when the target population was narrow and clear relative to other times.

SERVICE DEVELOPMENT FOR PEOPLE WITH SERIOUS MENTAL ILLNESS DURING THE PERIOD OF SYSTEM DEVELOPMENT

This chapter concludes, as did the previous one, with consideration of the fundamental service developments, which supported the process of deinstitutionalization and treatment of people with serious mental illness in the community.

Consider the example of James, age 21, another amalgamated, hypothetical case based on real patient records. After failing to make it in college, he lived with his parents. He fell ill with acute psychosis in 1993. His parents, strained by increasingly bizarre behavior at home, arranged for him to be brought the emergency room of the general hospital. James was hospitalized and remained there for six weeks. He was discharged to ambulatory care at the CMHC. He failed to connect with his clinicians and was readmitted, this time to the CMHC, for a brief, seven-day hospitalization before stepping down to partial hospital services, while living at home again. He was fortunate to be able to live at home with his parents, who nevertheless had been sorely strained by his behavior. His family entered a group that included other parents with ill family members in order to educate them about psychosis and to help them cope with their son. James resumed treatment on antipsychotic medicines and was assigned a case manager for the purpose of accessing services and benefits in the community. One service was psychosocial rehabilitation at a local community program, where he had an opportunity to learn and practice basic social skills. The case manager also helped him find vocational training and placement that permitted him to work part-time. As he stabilized, he was transferred into less intense, clinically led, group treatment, where his use of antipsychotic medicine was monitored. In the group, he shared his problems and set goals for himself along with others in similar circumstances. He relapsed and was hospitalized again for 10 days. On discharge, as his parents could no longer stand the strain on family life caused by his illness and as he preferred to find a place on his own, he was referred to a group residential care program. Clinical services were tightly linked to residential services by joint care planning on a special team at the mental health center. The same case manager that he had before was reactivated to help him make this transition to living in a group home.

While James's illness and treatment continued for many years with additional relapses, this account leaves him here, as his experience already illustrates the changes in access to services that had been achieved up to this time through the period of community services and system development. The contrast among the case examples at the end of chapter 4 and this one leads to appreciation of the change in services that occurred over this new period of public psychiatry. James's experience illustrates the accumulation of gains made in the modern era. It is important to note, however, that James's experience is rather simple compared to many of the people presenting for treatment at the CMHC by this time. Increasingly, people were presenting not with a single disorder but rather with co-occurring mental and substance-use problems, many of whom were embroiled with law enforcement for disorderly conduct or charges pending for drug use. In some cases, they were referred from court hearings in order to divert them from imprisonment into treatment. Furthermore, James was spared the indignity of homelessness, a social problem that was growing increasingly grave and prevalent among people with serious mental illness, a situation that enormously complicates clinical evaluation and treatment.

Table 5-2, which appeared in a first iteration in chapter 4, is repeated here in order to portray where services stood at the end of the period of community services and system development and the beginning of the next period of mainstreaming.

Additional service elements were still needed and remained as future tasks in order to care as effectively as possible for people with serious

Table 5-2 Service Type or Benefit by Period of Modern Public Psychiatry

Service Type or Benefit	Post–WW II	CMH	CSS
Asylum, chronic hospitalization	X		
Acute inpatient hospitalization		X	X
Partial hospitalization, intensive outpatient			X
Nursing home, long-term care		X	X
Routine outpatient, ambulatory care		X	X
Emergency room	X	X	X
Urgent care		X	X
Crisis intervention		X	X
Neighborhood clinics		X	
Prevention, early intervention		X	
Assertive community treatment			
Co-occurring services			
Vocational rehabilitation			X
Psychosocial rehabilitation	X		X
Case management, community support programs			X
Residential services			X
System development, local mental health authorities			X
Outreach to homeless			X
Recovery, quality of life goals			
Peer services			
Integrated primary medical care			
Medicaid Medicare		X	X
Supplemental Security Income Social Security Disability Insurance		X	X

Abbreviations: CMH, Community Mental Health; Post–WW II, Post–World War II.

mental illness in the community. The next chapter describes these developments during the period of mainstreaming at the CMHC.

CONCLUSION

The community mental health movement gave way to the period of community services and system development. In part, it did so as a function of the failure of the community mental health movement itself to meet the needs of people with chronic mental illness, who were being discharged from hospitals. Another factor in the change was a new political ideology that wanted the federal government out of the business of providing services. Under the new federalism, states now held the program initiative through state mental health authorities and state Medicaid plans. Economic recession added impetus to the transition. The new period, which focused on community services and system development in public psychiatry, was also one of evolution in terminology. The term public psychiatry slowly replaced community psychiatry as the means of referring to psychiatric practice in the public arena. The change in terminology was a function in part of the swing from federal to state support. During the new period, development in public psychiatry reoriented itself almost exclusively to care for chronically ill patients, who had been discharged from state hospitals into the community through special state and local systems of care.

Though the CMHC took steps in the new direction in public psychiatry, the institution did not move quickly or vigorously enough. The leadership of the CMHC adhered to a time-honored organizational structure designed to satisfy the demands of the state for services and to protect the academic programs of the YDP at the CMHC. A reorganization of the ambulatory services and academic programs was necessary in order to meet the new challenges in public sector patient care. Academic programs should have followed more the need and demand for services rather than academic standards dictating the services agenda and organization of the institution. Essentially, from 1982 to 1989, the CMHC fell behind developments in public psychiatry. Optimally, as an academic community mental health center, it should have been leading the way by embracing the change, evaluating the innovations, and making itself useful to the state DMH. The crisis in leadership at the CMHC in 1987 exposed, and added to, the lack of bold steps ahead during the evolution of public psychiatry in this period. The problems at the CMHC sorely tested the partnership between the state and the university. The difficulty of sustaining the CMHC with its tripartite multiple missions of service, education, and research, each complex in its own right, challenged the new leadership and the whole institution. By 1993, however, the CMHC had largely caught up to a changed service system in public psychiatry. At least, the troubles in leadership and management at the CMHC during the period of community services and system development were behind the institution.

Community services and system development in turn would be followed by a new phase of mainstreaming, the next major period of modern public psychiatry. It is interesting to ask what occasioned the transition from system development to mainstreaming. In part, it was a function of successful, piecemeal legislative advocacy regarding Medicaid after the revocation of the Mental Health Systems Act of 1980. This mainstreaming into Medicaid can be seen as a pilot study for Medicare and private insurers, though cost remained a huge hurdle. At the same time, there was no revival at a federal level of interest in expansion of special national initiatives, such as the community mental health movement. As a corollary, the federalism under the Reagan administration left program development in public psychiatry to decentralized state mental health agencies and state Medicaid plans. Perhaps most importantly, data from several services research studies did not support the value of system development. Two studies, a RWJ study and a joint RWJ/NIMH study, did not find that system development, in contrast to the availability of the services themselves, offered better clinical outcomes for individual patients. It is also true that states faced another fiscal crisis in the late stages of community services and system development, which was the latest in a series of budget crunches related to the economic cycle. The strategy of "medicaiding" mental health services became ever more attractive as a fiscal strategy for states. As a result, states increasingly partnered with the federal Center for Medicare and Medicaid Services in setting policy and system goals. Program development from state mental health authorities receded as a consequence. Mainstreaming, reflected in part by what was happening under Medicaid, became more prominent.

The Period of Mainstreaming and CMHC, 1993 to 2003

MAINSTREAMING

The next period of modern public psychiatry was mainstreaming of mental health benefits into general health and social programs. This period occurred in counterpoint to the "exceptionalism" policies of the previous two periods (Frank and Glied, 2006). The national health care debate of 1993 serves somewhat arbitrarily as a starting point for the purposes of this text. At that time, a mental health and substance-abuse work group cochaired by Tipper Gore, wife of Vice-president Al Gore, laid the groundwork during the unsuccessful legislative battle. That effort foreshadowed the goal of achieving nondiscriminatory health insurance benefits—such as equal deductibles, co-pays, and amount of service—for behavioral disorders as compared with other medical conditions (Grob and Goldman, 2007). Parity was the holy grail of mainstreaming. With significant victories along the way, it would take until 2008 to fully achieve this objective.

Despite an ominous beginning with repeal of the Mental Health Systems Act in 1981, the previous period in public psychiatry was notable for considerable policy and program advances for people with serious mental illness (Grob and Goldman, 2007). The Social Security Administration established new and fair rules for determination of psychosocial disability. Medicaid implemented reimbursement for several optional services of benefit to people with serious mental illness. Progress in residential services for people with psychosocial disabilities was substantial. Also, progress was made on discriminatory limits on Medicare insurance for certain psychiatric procedures. In a sense, the new period of mainstreaming was one of taking the policy and legislative strategies of the previous decade forward for all public and private payers for mental health services.

In order to achieve parity, two tasks were essential. One was to demonstrate the efficacy of psychiatric interventions; the other was to demonstrate a capacity to control costs through management of care.

With regard to the former, a surgeon general's report published in 1999 was a landmark publication that summarized the evidence for psychiatric interventions. With regard to the latter, managed behavioral health care entered the public sector. As private payers of health care services had done in the previous few years, public payers employed managed-care strategies to control their reimbursement costs. Managed care also made it possible for mental health system managers to reallocate costs to less expensive levels of care within the system of care. In Connecticut, by late in the decade, a threat of privatization under a conservative Republican governor loomed behind concerns about cost and the introduction of managed care.

MEDICAID

Depending on whether you emphasize the role of Medicaid in support of community-based services or Medicaid reimbursement as an example of mainstreaming, it is possible to bring Medicaid into the discussion in both the context of community services development and mainstreaming. Medicaid underwrote much of system development undertaken by states for people with serious mental illness. Medicaid also is a prime example of mainstreaming psychiatric entitlement benefits before the enactment of parity legislation in 2008. This text emphasizes the second point and continues a discussion of Medicaid in this chapter.

During the period of mainstreaming, the prominence of Medicaid as a payer for mental health services continued to grow. Shortly after the turn of the century, it was the single largest payer for behavioral services in the public sector. In Connecticut, as in other states according to varying time schedules, a subtle but real shift in policy initiative began to occur. On the one hand, were state mental health authorities, still largely preoccupied with community services and system development for people with serious mental illness. On the other, state Medicaid agencies were concerned about benefit definition, utilization management (UM), and reimbursement policies for mental health under Medicaid. Typically, the state Medicaid agencies had limited specialized mental health expertise. In Connecticut, this portrayal is only partially true. For example, the Department of Mental Health (DMH) held responsibility for state-administered general assistance to low income people and wrestled with the same questions as the state Medicaid agency for this portion of their services. Also, in contrast to other states the State of Connecticut was slow to pursue Medicaid matching reimbursement for mental health services. For example, Connecticut was the last state in the nation to seek reimbursement under the Medicaid Rehabilitation Option, and when it finally pursued this funding stream, it did so in a very limited way. Still, it is true that the State of Connecticut slowly and deliberately moved towards increasing Medicaid matching reimbursement by sequentially including specific services in its state plan, starting with Targeted Case Management, then mental health group homes, and with a 1915 (c) Waiver to support community-based services for people with mental illness being discharged from nursing homes.

THE CONNECTICUT MENTAL HEALTH CENTER IN 1993

While Medicaid, as a major and growing source of revenue, was driving the national development of services in a long-term perspective, the state general fund dollars supporting the state owned and operated CMHC served as a buffer against the need to turn to Medicaid to establish a revenue stream. Also, the State of Connecticut was slow to use Medicaid to fund state services. While revenues from Medicaid grew over time at the CMHC and made up 56% of total collections by 2005, these revenues went into the state general fund rather than contributing to the bottom line of the CMHC budget. It would be misleading, therefore, to say that the most salient feature of the two decades of community services development and mainstreaming at the CMHC, in particular, was Medicaid reimbursement for services, even as it may have been true for other, private, nonprofit, community mental health centers (Cutler et al., 2003).

For these reasons, the opening of a new period of public psychiatry was essentially imperceptible. It was appreciated best in retrospect. Of course, as the last chapter described, much was happening at the CMHC and added distractions were not sought. By 1993, the troubles of the crisis of leadership in 1987 and its aftermath were largely behind the institution. Leadership at the CMHC was stable. On a continuing basis, the CMHC needed to pay attention to the partnership that made up the institution. With regard to the Yale Department of Psychiatry (YDP), which was progressively biological and research oriented, it was important for the CMHC to represent the clinical mission of faculty staff members and to support career development for clinician-educators, who were essential for manning clinical services and management of the institution. With regard to the DMH, it was a time to strengthen the connection between academic programs and the state mission by making the academic programs indispensable in solving the policy, budgetary, and clinical challenges the DMH faced.

Established academic programs such as forensic psychiatry and substance abuse, which had been growing for decades, became centerpieces of the CMHC profile. New academic programs would emerge in recovery and medical psychiatry for integrating mental health and primary care, both of which would make essential contributions to the care of people with serious mental illness. A public health perspective on public psychiatry would once again prove useful in conceptualizing the field. These developments played out, not only during the period of mainstreaming, but also in the following period of transformation, which can be seen as a continuation of mainstreaming with shifting emphasis on certain elements.

To help orient the reader through this chapter, the major events and developments of the new period at the CMHC are summarized in the chronology provided in Table 6-1.

OUTREACH TO HOMELESS MENTALLY ILL PEOPLE

The next major element in the services spectrum at the CMHC was a program to provide outreach to mentally ill people who were

Table 6-1 Chronology at the CMHC During the Period of Mainstreaming, 1993-2003

1993	ACCESS program for homeless outreach begins
1993	CMHC Foundation begins
1994	ACT program begins at CMHC
1995	Residential services consolidated, first HUD grant
1995	CMHC co-occurring mental health and substance-abuse program begins
1995	A consolidated Department of Mental Health and Addiction Services
1996	New leadership at the CMHC (Jacobs)
1996	CMHC reorganizes into disorder-based, ambulatory clinical teams
1998	CMHC reorganization in response to public sector, managed care
1999	The Report on Mental Health of the U.S. Surgeon General
2000	New commissioner of Mental Health and Addiction Services (Kirk)
2001	IOM report on quality of medical care
2000	Program on Recovery and Community Health begins
2001	Peer services begin
2001	Disaster planning in response to terrorist attack
2001	Economic recession
2002	Integration of treatment and community-based services at CMHC

homeless. In response to a growing and unrelenting problem, the federal Substance Abuse Mental Health Administration funded demonstration projects for outreach. Faculty members at the CMHC were successful in competing as a site for the study, which was awarded in 1993. Known as Access to Community Care and Effective Services and Support (ACCESS), this program brought the CMHC once again into the cutting edge development of services for people who were seriously ill. Beginning in 1994, it offered outreach to homeless mentally ill people, a landmark new service element. Five years later, through the efforts of a local legislator, the state assembly voted on legislation to pick up the funding of homeless outreach, establishing it as a permanent element under a new name, the Outreach and Engagement Program, in the services offered at the CMHC. This program operated on the streets and under the bridges in order to engage homeless people. Often months were necessary to ultimately connect them to clinical services at the CMC.

THE CONNECTICUT MENTAL HEALTH CENTER FOUNDATION

In 1993, the CMHC Advisory Board, led by professor of law, Peter Shuck, and Robert Cole, the administrative director of the CMHC, took steps to incorporate the private, nonprofit Community Mental Health Center Foundation. Advisory board members thought it would be a good idea to have "friends of CMHC," who could raise money to pay for some of the things the state could not or would not pay for. Also, around the same time, Audrey Tyson, a psychiatric social worker, asked for permission to raise money to help patients be reestablished in the community after discharge from inpatient care. The Attorney General of Connecticut advised that a nonprofit organization would be the appropriate vehicle for fund-raising activities. Yale School of Law students, who staffed a nonprofit clinic of the school, provided legal advice and drafted documents of incorporation with the mission of improving the quality of life of the people served at the CMHC.

The initial goals for the foundation were quite modest. In a few years, the goals became more ambitious in concert with growing success in fund-raising from fashion shows, which became signature events, and more or less coincidentally with a substantial contribution from the estate of George Weltner, a medical sociologist, who took interest in the CMHC and its three-part mission. Consequently, the CMHC recruited and supported a part-time executive director to coordinate events and begin iterative processes of strategic planning. Over time, the foundation supported a variety of services and projects. These included, among others, "welcome baskets" for people leaving the hospital, who did not have the basic necessities to set up living independently; the support of social activities for people in treatment who were at risk for relapse, which led to successful competition for grant support; and wellness projects.

> Over time, the foundation supported a variety of services and projects.

Though no one foresaw it at the beginning, the foundation became a valuable vehicle for initiative and development outside the confines of state ownership and operation and of the YDP. This was true in the instance of nontraditional clinical services, such as fledgling recovery projects. It was also so with regard to start-up of pilot research, through active fund-raising and income from invested funds. Also, the foundation was an extremely useful tool for unifying the diverse groups of employees at the CMHC, and also for engaging the external community, where it became a effective private, nonprofit organization that forged partnerships with others. In these ways, the foundation contributed substantially to the services, academic missions, and the community relations of the CMHC, its parent institution.

ASSERTIVE COMMUNITY TREATMENT

In 1994, the CMHC implemented an assertive community treatment team (ACT). The creation of an ACT team can be seen as a residual task from the community services period. The DMH stimulated this program development in response to the initiatives of the program on chronic illness of the Robert Wood Johnson Foundation. It was late arriving at the CMHC, given the publication of evidence on ACT efficacy over 10 years earlier, but it was essential. ACT was designed for mentally ill people who were unable to keep appointments in a clinic and who frequently visited local emergency rooms, from which they were often hospitalized. ACT was a cornerstone of community services and system development for treatment in the community. The opportunity to provide these services to people with serious mental illness was a major new element in the local service system. The outpatient treatment teams of the CMHC remained intact.

By dint of sheer numbers and resources these teams remained the major ambulatory treatment component of the CMHC. The clinic-based teams functioned in communication with, but not integrated into, the novel community-based services. However, slowly but surely the service profile of the CMHC was changing. ACT joined ACCESS as novel service elements that established services outside the walls of the clinic and the hospital units at the CMHC. These clinical programs became a nexus for innovative program development over the next several years, in response to various federal and state funded initiatives to reach people with serious mental illness in the community, many of whom were homeless. They also brought in new kinds of medical and professional staff members. For example, one had anthropological expertise and eventually joined with recovery-oriented faculty members to provide an alternative to traditional clinic-based perspectives (Jacobs and Griffith, 2007).

RESIDENTIAL SERVICES

Starting in 1995, CMHC faculty members were instrumental in competing for federal Housing and Urban Development grants to establish supportive housing in the community. As noted in the previous chapter, a place of residence became a critical element in plans of care for many people with serious mental illness, in part because of the absence of affordable housing in the community. Indeed, over time, as states faced repeated budget crises and retrenched on hospital-based services, leaving that to general hospitals, residential placements promised to become an essential platform for treating chronically ill and disabled people in the community. Professional staff at the CMHC engaged with others in the service system of community mental health providers and the city to address the shortage of housing resources for this target population. Over the years, CMHC faculty staff members cochaired a citywide consortium to conduct censuses of the homeless, assess needs, and collaborate on annual grants for additional services. Section 8 funding for people with disabilities supplemented the supportive housing program. Both of these federal sources supplemented investments made in residential placements by the DMH with general fund dollars. The annual grant-writing efforts of the Continuum, coled by the CMHC, was substantial. It amounted to an additional support for residential placements of over $30 million over the next 13 years.

As a final note, residential resources were an essential platform for community-based care. At the CMHC, public management of residential resources created an alternative to hospital-based services that had originally defined it as a hospital. When managed care arrived in public psychiatry during the period of mainstreaming, a residential base became even more important. As later chapters will describe, given a shortage of resources for acute hospital care in psychiatry, residential services would become a fundamental platform for clinical services managed by public psychiatry in the community.

DISORDER-BASED CLINICAL TEAMS

Clinical programs in the institutions of the YDP, starting at the West Haven Veteran's Medical Center, moved to disorder-based teams. The CMHC decided to follow suit and started planning in 1995, finally implementing disorder-based teams on the ambulatory clinical services in fall, 1996. The three traditional ambulatory treatment teams reconstituted themselves as: a team for psychotic disorders, one for mood disorders, and a third for anxiety disorders, traumatic disorders, and personality disorders. As comorbidity was common in the treated population, skepticism persisted about the specificity of treatments for particular disorders. As a result, some clinicians were reluctant to move in this direction at the CMHC. Also, the change was a departure from the time-honored, homogenized ambulatory teams, on which psychotherapy was the cornerstone of care.

There were multiple rationales for persisting in the change. Disorder-based teams were in part a response to the success of biologic treatment models of the time, as well as to the development of specific psychotherapies for certain disorders. The new disorder-based teams were predicated on the assumption that enough specialized knowledge of interventions was disorder-based and justified specialization within ambulatory services, as opposed to everyone being a generalist. It also made sense in light of a progressive emphasis on evidence-based treatment. Further, it made sense as a platform for clinical research. Finally, it made sense as the reimbursement policies of federal entitlement programs were predicated on a medical model, and managed care strategies played out within the framework of a medical model. Going forward, the disorder-based teams offered an opportunity to concentrate expertise in diagnosis and treatment and better keep up with new evidence-based developments.

Residential programs and the ACT team were exceptions to the diagnosis-based reorganization. Group and family programs at the CMHC were lost as organizational units as a result of this disorder-based organization. Also, the final vestiges of a psychotherapy model in ambulatory care, which prevailed over 30 years, dissipated at the CMHC. The segregation of care of the chronically ill ended. By 1996, the chronically ill were mainstreamed completely into disorder-based teams. It was a good example of how centralized YDP initiatives, under a new deputy chair, were driving developments at the CMHC during this time.

Reorganization into disorder-based teams placed the mental health teams at the CMHC on a more equal footing with substance-use treatment, which had grown in importance. Of overriding importance, the substance-use treatment team was probably the strongest example in the

CMHC of a clinical team that integrated the three missions of service, clinical research, and education on a team level. As an alternative to understanding addictions as a moral or ethical problem, and also as biological studies established the brain mechanisms of addiction, substance-use professionals were pursuing a medical model for substance-use disorders. In order to improve integration of the missions for all the clinical teams and take advantage of biomedical developments, the success of the substance-use disorders model seemed to make sense.

COMORBIDITY: MENTAL ILLNESS, AND SUBSTANCE USE

More or less coincidentally, the disorder-based reorganization of the mental health teams occurred when the CMHC was evolving in its approach to treating comorbid, mental illness and substance-use disorders. The disorder-based teams provided a foundation for addressing the conspicuous problem of comorbidity in the patient population. Striving for a combination and integration of the two clinical models of mental health and substance use became a long-term, institutional goal. The strategy at first, in 1995, was to develop a special treatment team for co-occurring disorders. The team was pulled together from within the existing resources of the CMHC. The implementation of the co-occurring disorders team was a harbinger of a trend. As the numbers of applicants for treatment with co-occurring disorders continued to grow and eventually surpass 50% and as comorbid patients repeatedly fell in the cracks between the specialized substance-use treatment team and the mental health treatment teams, the CMHC set a goal for all its clinicians to become dually competent. Over time, the CMHC adopted a variety of educational, supervisory and, to some extent, recruitment strategies to achieve this goal, which yet remains a challenging but never fully achieved ideal.

A DEPARTMENT OF MENTAL HEALTH AND ADDICTION SERVICES

In 1995, the Connecticut DMH incorporated the Connecticut Alcohol and Drug Addiction Commission and became the Department of Mental Health and Addiction Services (DMHAS). This reorganization of state agencies was of little or no consequence for the CMHC. This was so because the administrative structure of the combined state organizational structure remained for several more years essentially two silos of service. The reasons for the division lay in the separate histories of the two sectors of service. Local mental heath authorities, serving as intermediaries between independent agencies and the DMHAS, had already brought system development on the mental health side. Substance-use agencies operated independently, related directly to the DMHAS, and wanted to keep it that way. Substance-use services had split off from mental health 25 years before in order to foster growth and development. The overall size of the substance-use services still remained smaller than mental health, though a number of individual agencies were larger than their mental health counterparts. Many of the more entrepreneurial substance-use agency heads still remained in leadership. They feared they would not fare as well in integrated systems.

MANAGED CARE AND NEW LEADERSHIP FOR THE CMHC

In 1996, Dr. Selby Jacobs, a public health psychiatrist, was appointed director of the CMHC. The CMHC was beginning to address the challenges of managed care, which was one of the manifestations of mainstreaming in public psychiatry.

After several years of growth in the private sector of psychiatry, managed care arrived in force in public psychiatry in Connecticut. Under the assumptions of managed care, the reorientation of thinking in the public sector of psychiatry was enormous. The background for managing care was no longer mental health systems or clinical theory but rather corporate organization, economic theory, and marketplace dynamics. Both federal and state governments were focused on economic variables, such as cost, value, and incentives, to shape the health and mental health care systems. At its best, a focus on value brought into consideration not only cost but also efficacy of treatment as the two factors in the equation of value ($v = e/c$). Underlying this approach was a federal and state attitude that government should be minimally involved in providing health care, if at all.

Privatization of behavioral health services, though it never materialized at this point in Connecticut, was a background theme much talked about in the state under a conservative governor. State budget crises, which aggravated after 2000, fueled the talk. It was known that managed care as a UM and cost control mechanism played itself out in the private sector after wringing the high costs of hospital care out of the system. Privatization was a logical next step for state operated services.

> Privatization was a logical next step for state-operated services.

In 1997, the DMHAS launched the development of integrated service systems (ISS) in response to the prospect of managed care and privatization in the public psychiatry. The process included 6 state owned and operated community mental health centers, 17 private nonprofit centers, and all the independent, private nonprofit substance-use agencies in the state. The goal was to better integrate care, including mental health and substance-abuse services, and to control costs. As a reflection of the new business thinking, directors of state facilities were now called chief executive officers. Consultants introduced a new system model with multiple levels of care designed to be responsive to the demands of managed care tactics to control costs. Business plans and models of care, including incentives, productivity, and value, were under discussion, as opposed to traditional public mental health systems.

The ISS process challenged the old community-support program models established in the previous period of public sector services. In the process, competition and conflict arose among private nonprofit agencies, which saw themselves as more efficient and innovative, and state owned facilities such as the CMHC. Though building on the community support program model in many ways, as had private sector behavioral health care, the ISS deliberations essentially offered a conceptual alternative to it. After two years and innumerable meetings, the ISS process collapsed. It sank on the shoals of resistance from substance-use agencies to accept local system integration with mental health, which was already organized into local mental health authorities.

LEVELS OF CARE

At the CMHC, a strategic planning process translated into efforts to make clinical services managed-care ready. Given that managed care focused on hospital inpatient services as the high payoff, low-hanging fruit for cost control, the CMHC addressed hospital length of stay as a priority. As a result, lengths of stay on the acute inpatient unit of the CMHC reached 9 days by 1999, having been close to 30 days only 10 years before. In order to shorten lengths of stay in the hospital, it was necessary to have lower levels of care for step-down of patient care. These levels of care needed to extend beyond acute care, which was within the walls of the institution, to multiple, ambulatory, community-based interventions, as well as support services in order to manage seriously ill patients outside of the hospital in the community. As a result of community services development of the previous period in public psychiatry, many of these levels of care and support services had accumulated over previous years.

However, it was necessary to conceptualize and integrate them into a continuum supporting short hospital stays. The CMHC, as a result of these efforts, reinforced several levels of care such as intensive outpatient, and community services such as case management, assertive treatment, and outreach.

A basic premise in this regard was the idea that ambulatory services were the foundation, including multiple levels of care, and crisis and outreach services. This was a departure from a long-standing premise that hospital beds were the main platform from which the CMHC offered services. Indeed, the hospital platform was shrinking in number of beds, and residential services promised to be the platform for long-term and acute care in the future in the public sector. In this way, the identity of the CMHC continued to evolve in the direction already set by changes under community services and system development, the previous period of public psychiatry.

ADMINISTRATIVE AND CLINICAL REORGANIZATION AT THE CMHC

In response to the challenge of managed care and statewide ISS planning, the CMHC administratively reorganized along the lines of a general hospital. A general hospital model was time-honored, flatter than existing CMHC structures, and more efficient in use of professional manpower and for communication. The new model contrasted with a residual academic leadership model, which persisted from the opening of he CMHC. Under managed care, it was necessary to demonstrate that the CMHC could be as flat, lean, and efficient as its private nonprofit peers, or at least more efficient than it had been previously. Actually, there had been progressive erosion of administrative resources at the CMHC over the years as a result of unrelenting fiscal pressures. In a sense, the CMHC made a virtue of necessity. The main resistance to reorganization was from those at middle management levels, often physicians, who lost administrative power. For the most part, other clinicians embraced the change, as it ultimately was less hierarchical, more professionally democratic, and more open for communication among leadership, professional staff, and team-based clinicians.

The reorganization aimed for a lean, flat, administrative structure that made efficient use of high-cost professionals. For example, the leadership eliminated division chiefs and required clinical units to report directly to a director of clinical services. The reorganization freed faculty member physicians from administrative tasks and established them as attending physicians or program directors on the inpatient and outpatient teams. They reported to a medical director in senior leadership, through a medical and professional staff structure. In this case, the goal was to enable physicians to pursue clinical or academic rather than administrative tasks.

Internal utilization management (UM) was another part of reorganization to ensure that CMHC services conformed to the expectations of payers in the public arena that now were managing care. The CMHC established independent internal UM in order to focus the clinical services on the need for change and to bring it about. At the same time, because it was an internal process, the CMHC was able to evaluate and adjust the system if one side of the institution—for instance, UM—was doing too much damage to the other side, such as clinical services. The CMHC adjusted levels of care based on utilization data and on the constraints of reimbursement policies employed by government entitlements in order to control costs. Nagging scarcity of resources also served as a constraint.

It is interesting how this reorganization, occasioned by a need to operate under managed care, bridged back to medical concepts of institutional organization of the community mental health movement and before. The CMHC had been through a major crisis in leadership and a period where it had lagged in following changes in public psychiatry as it developed community services and systems for people with serious mental illness. At that point in time, the bias in institutional identity as a hospital, to some extent written into the original memorandum of agreement between the state and university partners, prevented a nimble turn toward identification with rehabilitative tasks and extension into the community. Going forward during mainstreaming, the preservation of a latent hospital identity over the years—reinforced by three-year JCAHO site visits under hospital standards, a choice made in 1984—served the institution well. Even later, in the period of transformation, the priority to integrate primary care and mental health in order to address the shortened life expectancy of people with serious mental illness fit well into the new structure.

The reorganization was a local example of how, though building on community services implemented in the previous period, payers and their managed care strategies (in other words mainstreaming) were now driving program initiative. In the previous period in public psychiatry, the proximate agent of change was the state mental authority. Now, initiative was shifting from state departments of mental health to payers for service in the public arena, such as Medicaid, state Medicaid agencies, and the behavioral managed care organizations subcontracted to control costs (Buck, 2003).

PRODUCTIVITY

A nagging problem at the CMHC was abysmally low productivity of clinicians. The institution developed a definition of productivity as the percentage of work hours spent in face-to-face contact with recipients of care. It took a few months just to reach a mutually agreed-on definition, which was part of the process. The standard of the DMHAS in an old commissioner's policy was 50%. Productivity at the CMHC averaged 27%. This performance was better than the sister state owned institutions of the CMHC. The CMHC leadership believed it was necessary to take on this issue to assure the public, the conservative state government (antagonistic to an academic institution), and its private, nonprofit competitive agencies (which were touting their efficiency), that the CMHC could husband resources effectively. An institutional focus on productivity served the purpose of demonstrating a commitment to efficiency and value. It may be an unusual way to think for public institutions, but these were new times.

For many reasons, the CMHC never did get average productivity much above 35%. Still, the attention the institution paid to the problem put it out in front of its sister state institutions. It also took some of the edge off the attacks on it as an academic institution. In the end, the academic CMHC was just as productive, or more so, than its sister institutions. However, it never achieved a level of productivity that was competitive with private sector performance.

BUDGET CRISES AND FISCAL PRESSURE

By 1999, there were budget deficits at the CMHC. Within a year there were state budget deficits as part of a national economic recession of 2000-01. The only exceptions to budget stringency were for court-mandated categorical funding or federal grant programs. The CMHC entered a period of perennial hiring freezes, which created a plateau of clinical staff and programs and, indeed, some shrinkage of general clinical services. This resulted in tension between the CMHC and the DMHAS for a few years. The challenge for the CMHC leadership was to find ways to innovate and maintain a balanced, reasonably comprehensive range of services under this fiscal pressure. This time was essentially a continuation of fiscal pressure discussed and documented in the previous chapter. By 2001, the Connecticut Office of Policy and Management, the governor's budget office, began to target research at the center for budget cuts. To defend itself, the CMHC renewed its commitment to a three-part mission, which was considered not only a unique aspect but also strength of the institution. The basic tenet of the institution was that the three missions, including clinical services, teaching, and research, enhanced each other. Essentially, the position of CMHC was: all the missions or none.

In retrospect, the arrival of managed care in the public sector of services in Connecticut signaled that the CMHC was in a prolonged budget-cutting phase of institutional life. This period of time, especially

> The three missions—clinical services, teaching, and research—enhanced each other.

after 1999, appears as one of managing downsizing while dealing with repeated budget deficits. The institutional coping strategy included flattening of administrative structures, stretching clinician-to-patient ratios, and retrenchment in some programs. It was management of scarcity in resources while setting and maintaining quality standards and striving for innovation within existing resources by emphasizing priorities and balance in programs.

THE SEEDS OF ANOTHER BUILDING ADDITION TO THE CMHC

In the midst of these administrative challenges for the CMHC, by 1998, the Ribicoff Research Facility, under the leadership of Dr. Eric Nestler, had built an enduring reputation as one of the leading neurobiological research facilities in the United States. This fact was not lost on the dean of Yale School of Medicine (YSM). The dean made a commitment to expand research facilities for Dr. Nestler and his colleagues at the CMHC. He generously recognized this commitment as an opportunity to engage the university and the State of Connecticut once again in a joint construction project. The commissioner of the DMHAS agreed in principle. The New Haven legislative delegation to the Connecticut Assembly, under the leadership of assembly member Patricia Dillon, appropriated $5 million to approximately match the YSM commitment. Design began, but the project was fraught with conflict over leasing, by wavering commitment on the university side, and by delays. There were many opportunities for discouragement and failure. The commitment of CMHC administration to working out the obstacles finally led to success. It took 11 years to bring this project to fruition and finally dedicate the building in 2009. Tortuous though it was, the process of planning served to periodically reinforce the commitment of the two partners to the CMHC enterprise.

TREATMENT AND REHABILITATION

Much service development had happened at the CMHC during the previous period of public psychiatry, including the creation of a local mental health authority (LMHA) in a system of community-based rehabilitative services for individuals with serious mental illness. In addition, there were new special services, such as ACT, case management, outreach to homeless mentally ill people, and supportive residential services.

A challenge for the CMHC was to integrate treatment and rehabilitation was both professional and institutional. Unfortunately, with a few exceptions psychiatrists at the CMHC and in the YDP had lost touch with the professional responsibility for the disabilities associated with chronic mental illness. With the exception of the American Association of Community Psychiatrists and a small number of subspecialist public psychiatrists across the country, rehabilitation had essentially become a nonmedical professional domain in the community. Interprofessional rivalries aggravated the gap opened between treatment and rehabilitation. These facts stood in contrast to the traditional state hospitals before community mental health, where rehabilitation was part of overall plans of care under a treatment plan ordered by the hospital physician. Thus, part of a broader clinical challenge for the CMHC was to reintegrate disabilities and rehabilitative interventions back into comprehensive plans of care by physicians for individuals in treatment. To achieve this goal, the CMHC needed to invigorate professional roles for physicians by expanding them to include rehabilitative tasks as essential part of plans of care.

Organizational arrangements at the CMHC aggravated the division between treatment and rehabilitation. The community-based rehabilitative and support services through the LMHA were administratively separate from ambulatory clinical services. Despite efforts at communication and coordination, administrative boundaries went up between clinical services and the community. Also, the separate management of residential resources at the CMHC aggravated the problem. These boundaries were a problem, which had to be solved not only to integrate treatment and rehabilitation but also as the CMHC developed short lengths of stay and multiple levels of care in the circumstances of shrinking resources. Stemming from the ISS planning process, it is also true that the DMHAS requested the CMHC to integrate the management of all its institutional and community-based resources under the LMHA.

The CMHC decided to establish a unified leadership for all these programs. Also, the institution undertook the long-term task of bringing together clinical treatment and rehabilitation in comprehensive plans of care for individual patients. As an outgrowth of this process of change, the CMHC later integrated employment specialists—employees of community-based rehabilitation agencies—into its clinical teams. The integration on a leadership level led to multiple performance-improvement goals for the institution, such as combined CMHC and community strategic planning, and eventually a recovery strategic plan. Also, these changes progressively integrated clinic-based functions into the community, lowering—if not breaking down—the remaining walls of the hospital. Finally, it should be noted that the integration of treatment services and rehabilitation can be seen in part as a function of the emerging recovery movement.

THE RECOVERY MOVEMENT

Culminating a movement that had developed over 20 years and which established a legal basis for patients' rights and empowerment, the Americans with Disabilities Act (ADA) of 1990 created national antidiscrimination regulations in employment, accommodations, telecommunications, and transportation. It made it all the more important for mental health professionals to pay attention to residential and rehabilitative resources as essential building blocks of the ambulatory environment of ambulatory care. The act was also major landmark in mainstream legislative successes subsequent to the repeal of the MHSA in 1982.

The recovery movement developed as the vehicle for pursuing the rights and empowerment of people with mental illness. In the words of the 1999 surgeon general's report, recovery is the notion that "a person with mental illness can recover even though the illness is not cured," and "is a way of living a satisfying, hopeful, and contributing life even with the limitations caused by illness." The recovery movement was both indigenous to psychiatry and part of a mainstream movement toward ownership and consumerism in health and welfare policy. In this sense, it was yet another example of mainstreaming of mental health care.

Recovery began in earnest at the CMHC about the year 2000 and became a powerful agent of change. The recovery movement challenged the CMHC to give full attention to involvement of recipients of care into all levels of the institution, from governance down to clinical practice. Over the next few years, the role of recipients of care grew through special initiatives to enhance their preparation for board roles, support roles in the emergency room and urgent care services, advisory roles regarding recovery on the inpatient units, and roles in wellness and disease management. With the guidance of consumer leadership, the CMHC referred to recipients of care as peers, an improvement in terminology over business inspired terms such as consumers and clients, but still not perfect. On a clinical level, the tool for introduction of recovery into the CMHC was person-centered care, described further in the next chapter.

The momentum generated in the CMHC for recovery added to efforts to evolve an academic program on serious and persistent mental illness, which had begun 15 years before. The crisis in leadership in 1987 had most damaged clinical research, which was not identified with neuroscience or addictions or forensic psychiatry. This was true insofar as service and state agency demands for service development kept clinical research unsettled. As a product of the recovery movement at the CMHC, a new academic program, Recovery and Community Health, emerged in 2000 under the leadership of Dr. Larry Davidson and colleagues. In subsequent years, CMHC faculty members helped to put the DMHAS on the map as the "recovery state" and became an important bridging structure to the department. With recovery as a building block and a growing cadre of clinician investigators on the ambulatory treatment teams of the CMHC, a successful R25 research education grant application organized many of the clinical faculty around clinical research on serious mental illness. This educational vehicle pulled together a broad range of faculty staff members into a coherent clinical, teaching, and research program. In part, its success emphasized that the CMHC was firmly committed to preserving a focus on chronic mental illness despite a progressive change in character of the target population served by public psychiatry in Connecticut. Later, in the period of transformation, the challenge of addressing the shortened life expectancy of people with serious mental illness would galvanize this academic center again.

> The CMHC was firmly committed to preserving a focus on chronic mental illness.

The recovery movement also ought to be seen as part of mainstreaming, though not in its origins. For example, once it was underway, payers quickly appreciated how they could take advantage of recovery ideas as part of a larger, mainstream development of consumerism in medicine. Under the Bush administration, this appropriation fit into a political philosophy of ownership. The point about recovery as a mainstream phenomenon is important in order to understand some of the momentum behind the concept of recovery. It is an example of how payers can insert financing strategies into otherwise ideological, professional, and progressively evidence-based developments.

THE SURGEON GENERAL'S REPORT

The 1999 Report on Mental Health by the Surgeon General of the United States Public Health Service was the first ever of its kind (USDHHS, 1999). It reviewed the existing evidence for the efficacy of psychiatric interventions, thereby heralding the evidence base of psychiatric practice. It recommended better dissemination of evidence-based treatments. Returning to a foundational idea of the community mental health movement, it placed mental health policy in a public health context, a perspective that had been lost in the period of community services and system development for chronic illness, and during the early years of mainstreaming. It foreshadowed the New Freedom Commission of 2003, which called for early detection, early intervention, and prevention. It highlighted the idea of burden of disease, which introduced not only the concept but also a metric based on indirect assessment of disability combined with mortality data. Analyses of burden of disease established a high priority for mental health in mainstream public health (Murray and Lopez, 1996). In all these ways, the surgeon general's report reinforced the idea of psychiatry as a part of medicine and advanced the agenda of mainstreaming. As the surgeon general said in his introduction to the report, "There is no health without mental health."

In its recommendations, the report also asserted that diagnosis and treatment must be "tailored to individual circumstances," while taking into consideration age, sex, race, culture, and other factors that shape personal identity. Another, later, report of the surgeon general in 2001 on disparities in mental health outcomes for representatives of ethnic minorities reinforced the agenda of cultural competence as a foundation for increasing access and reducing disparities in outcomes (USDHHS, 2001).

The CMHC used the report of the surgeon general to reinforce multiple areas of knowledge and practice. This chapter and the next document many of these initiatives. For the sake of demonstrating the far-reaching implications of the report, it is useful to list them here. They include: a more aggressive introduction of best practices; the translation into practice of discoveries from research, both in the institution and reported in the literature; the introduction of computer supported, evidence-based medicine into education programs; progress in programs of recovery and serious mental illness; patient-centered care, which came later as part of a successful grant application; early intervention in high-risk syndromes and initial psychotic illness; and renewed commitment, through cultural competence, to serving representatives of ethnic and racial minorities, a focus that had been sidelined within the institution with the closure of the HWH Division at the end of the community mental health era.

QUALITY OF CARE AND MEASUREMENT OF OUTCOMES

The Institute of Medicine (IOM) published a report on deaths from medical error in hospitals in 1999, estimating that up to 98,000 deaths resulted annually from mistakes in practice. In 2001, an IOM report appeared, entitled "Crossing the Quality Chasm." This report set an agenda, for all of medicine, to attend to outcomes of care. It offered an alternative vision to managed care, which, despite the rhetoric about quality, was focused mainly on cost reduction. The quality agenda was just as important for public psychiatry as for any other part of medicine, particularly under the assumptions of mainstreaming during this period. Under pay-for-performance policies, payers began to introduce outcome measures as a way of shaping how clinicians practiced. Regulatory agencies, such as the Joint Commission on Accreditation of Health Organizations (JCAHO), picked up the issue of patient safety and incorporated such goals into regulatory review standards.

Stemming from the IOM report, approaches to patient safety began to incorporate systems perspectives to complement the individual professional responsibility of physicians and other professionals. The report laid out an agenda for improving patient safety based on the model of large-scale, high-risk industrial and commercial enterprises such as airlines. A system perspective represented a fundamental change in the philosophy underlying quality control, from one of striving for perfection, a traditional and typical attitude inculcated in medical schools, to one of accepting that mistakes and errors occur, learning from them, and designing procedures to avoid or minimize them. Patient safety shifted to being primarily a collective, system problem rather than a personal professional one, though elements of both perspectives had been present before and after the report.

The CMHC believed that the quality agenda was a major new direction in development of services—and certainly for regulatory review. From this point forward, in preparation for JCAHO site visits every three years, the institution, building on quality improvement processes introduced eight years earlier, incorporated specific goals into its institutional performance. Examples include medication reconciliation when patients moved from service to service, and reduction in use of seclusion and restraints, one of the highest-risk procedures in behavioral health. Under the leadership of the CMHC medical director, medical and professional staff confronted the potential conflict between professional personal responsibilities and a system approach to safety in incident reviews of adverse occurrences in patient care.

A NEW COMMISSIONER OF MENTAL HEALTH AND ADDICTION SERVICES

In 2000, the governor appointed, as the new commissioner of the DMHAS, Dr. Thomas Kirk, an addictions expert and deputy commissioner under the incumbent. The appointment of a new commissioner, offered an opportunity for the CMHC to renew and rebuild a relationship with the commissioner and his state agency.

The CMHC leadership believed that the institution had to demonstrate its usefulness to the DMHAS. This strategy was more fundamental than it might appear at first glance. It moved beyond the time-honored institutional strategy of earlier periods of playing the university off against the state, and vice versa. This strategy had been predicated on the assumption that such dynamics helped to sustain an independent and academic agenda for the CMHC. In the traditional formulation, educational and research agendas could trump the demands of service development. In the new view, education and, to the extent possible, research ought to follow the rapidly changing agenda in public services, which was being driven by budget deficits, consumerism, mainstreaming, quality, value, and productivity. The old view had been part of the problem leading up to the crisis in leadership in 1987. The CMHC had indeed strayed too far from its own understanding of "political economics" and systems theory. With the appointment of a new commissioner in 2000, the leadership of the center set out to make a fresh start.

The CMHC engaged DMHAS in every way it could, ranging from prevention to co-occurring disorders, chronic mental illness, gambling, medical care of people with serious mental illness, recovery, forensics, and manpower training. The two areas that were particularly fruitful were the development of recovery in the state agency, where a CMHC faculty member was instrumental in getting DMHAS started, and forensic psychiatry, building on a long-standing relationship that had begun in 1979 and had helped the DMHAS build its own forensic capacity. By making the CMHC faculty members useful as consultants on key policy issues or problems, the CMHC demonstrated the value of an academic community mental health center in the statewide system. This value routinely encompassed policy and clinical domains, but also served to provide political cover for DMHAS when, for example, forensic experts of the CMHC provided consultation on high-profile or high-risk forensic patients being evaluated and treated by DMHAS.

Over the next few years, the DMHAS established a national reputation in the areas of recovery, co-occurring disorders, and transformation. In addition, during the tenure of the new commissioner, the National Alliance on Mental Illness (NAMI) awarded high marks to the DMHAS for the quality and responsiveness of its public sector service system.

> The DMHAS established a national reputation in the areas of recovery, co-occurring disorders, and transformation.

DISASTER READINESS

While multiple developments were unfolding—subsumed under the rubric of mainstreaming—the agenda for public psychiatry suddenly expanded. On September 11, 2001, terrorists attacked the World Trade Center in Manhattan and altered American attitudes forever. In response to this horrifying event, the CMHC played an active role in offering triage, counseling, and crisis services to victims of the attack, who were evacuated from Manhattan through New Haven. Part of the agenda for American society after the attack was to develop disaster plans to cope in the event of another attack. The DMHAS took part in statewide planning for disaster relief. The DMHAS and its sister agency, the Department of Children and Families, took the initiative in developing a disaster behavioral-health response plan and in organizing and training disaster response teams. These efforts were assisted by psychological trauma experts from Yale University and the University of Connecticut, and were coordinated with the work of other state agencies.

As a facility of the DMHAS, the CMHC participated in the planning and figured in the plan. In addition, the CMHC participated in citywide planning in order to coordinate a local response. Among other things, the CMHC designated crisis intervention teams, formulated plans for operating a large facility in the event of a disaster, and laid plans for the care of the most acutely ill psychiatric patients in the community in such conditions. In this way, the terrorist attack of September 11th introduced an entirely new agenda into the life of the institution. More recent examples of contingency planning were the preparations required for epidemics of bird (H5N1) and swine (H1N1) influenza, in which waves of acute illness among patients and staff members and absenteeism among affected staff would pose challenges.

EVOLUTION OF A MEDICAL MODEL FOR PUBLIC PSYCHIATRY AT THE CMHC

Throughout its history, public psychiatry has needed a robust model for conceptualizing the care it provides to its target populations. Perhaps, under the assumptions of mainstreaming, public psychiatry needs such a model more than ever. This section argues that a broad medical model would serve this purpose well. Recovery or system models exist as alternate candidates for model building. Neither of these inherently accommodates medical roles and tasks, nor are they as broad as models available in medicine. Consumer models of care are also possible choices. Person-centered care is the best example of a model that is an evidence-based practice and serves to connect the individual who has an illness to an array of medical and social services. Person-centered care integrates well with a broad medical model for psychiatric practice.

Earlier in modern public psychiatry, during the community mental health movement, a medical model prevailed that incorporated public health and preventive perspectives. During community services and system development, psychiatrists and the models they used to conceptualize treatment did not fare well. It was almost as if there was an implicit assumption that the "system" and system managers would take care of the patients. Without evidence that systems added value to patient outcomes, given the absence of a special and benevolent system, and under the assumptions of mainstreaming, it became essential again to formulate a clinical model that supported a comprehensive, multidisciplinary plan of care for individuals.

A model is not only important for organization of clinical care, it is also important for orientation and development of the profession. In the large interdisciplinary field of public psychiatry—including psychiatric social workers, psychologists, and masters level business managers, some of whom are competing for leadership—it is useful for psychiatrists to have a conceptual model for organizing the multiple challenges and forces shaping the public system. In order to meet the full range of needs of the people served by public psychiatry, the times called for a biological, psychological, and social clinical model that incorporated public health and rehabilitative tasks.

> A conceptual model organizes the multiple challenges and forces shaping the public system.

It is also important to appreciate how payers for services also figured in the choice of model. For example, one implication of Medicaid reimbursement was its construction on a medical model. Thus, reinforcement of a medical model was one of the consequences of mainstreaming mental health benefits under Medicaid. Medicaid was a harbinger of things to come. Medicare, the other major federal entitlement, also built its reimbursement on medial models, as did private insurers. To obtain reimbursement, it was necessary to establish medical necessity, which was predicated generally on a physician's order for treatment of an acute illness. By the way, Medicaid was a good role model for other payers insofar as it did not discriminate against people with psychiatric disorders in its benefits, deductibles, and co-pays. When managed care arrived in Medicaid, behavioral carve-outs were the rule, though all of medical care was managed. The implicit incorporation of a medical model into

Medicaid, as well as the reimbursement policies of other payers, served to underscore the role of psychiatrists in mental health care. It added impetus to consideration of medical models for public practice.

Though many psychiatrists consider continuous quality improvement an annoying added task on top of busy clinical schedules, the quality agenda in modern medicine and public psychiatry serves as an antidote to concerns about cost pursued primarily by payers. It is also interesting to note how the IOM formulated and led the quality agenda. In psychiatry, quality assurance procedures made essential contributions to improving the clinical management of poly-pharmaceutical treatment and to reducing the use of high-risk restraints and seclusion to manage threatening behavior. These are examples of how organized medicine can set policy agendas of fundamental importance to public practice.

Beyond the issues already discussed, several other factors during the period of mainstreaming in public psychiatry reinforced a medical model in public psychiatry. At the CMHC, these included evidence-based medicine, translation of discoveries and best practices, disorder-based teams, and revitalized public health efforts stemming from the report of the surgeon general. These factors and processes stemming from them unfolded rapidly over a few years. They reinforced the need and the value of a broad medical model for conceptualizing the work of the CMHC.

Despite some misgivings, which arose during the previous period of system development (see Chapter 5), a broad medical model has served the CMHC well during mainstreaming, and over most of its history. For contemporary purposes, it is possible to broaden a narrow biomedical model that is typically associated with much of practice during the rise of biological psychiatry, by using it as a base. A broad medical model attends to biological, psychological, and social manifestations of illness and incorporates public health, as well as the spectrum of chronic illness, disability, rehabilitation and recovery. Though a medical emphasis is prominent in this iteration, reflecting the times, it is a reincarnation of the biopsychosocial model, which psychosomatic psychiatrists defined for psychiatry when biological psychiatry began to ascend. Such a model attends to biological, psychological, and social manifestations of illness and incorporates public health as well as the spectrum of chronic illness, disability, rehabilitation, and recovery. It supports public psychiatry in its core responsibility: serving people with serious mental illness.

Finally, it is important to appreciate that a strong tradition of medical science, including clinical and chronic disease epidemiology and services research, is in place to support a broad medical model. Scientific inquiry serves the purpose of evaluating clinical insights and putting them in perspective. It supports understanding of the etiology, nature, and treatment of psychiatric disorders. A scientific base roots the practice and services of public psychiatry in evidence. Evidence provides a basis for making choices about practice and provides by a process of evaluation. Also, public health and epidemiology bring a population perspective to heath care, which supplements clinical views derived from serving individuals in offices, clinics, and labs. The two views are complementary and additive. Knowledge of the status and dynamics of diseases in the community challenges narrow clinical views and the limits of clinical science. The combination of clinical and social sciences suggests an agenda, not only for practice, but also for use of resources and scientific inquiry. In summary, science and complementary scientific disciplines, in contrast to often-competitive political and ideological movements, provide methods for progress through evidence-based evaluation and practice.

SERVICE DEVELOPMENT FOR PEOPLE WITH SERIOUS MENTAL ILLNESS DURING THE PERIOD OF MAINSTREAMING

As in the previous two chapters, we conclude with consideration of the service developments that support the process of deinstitutionalization and care for people with serious mental illness in the community. As noted before, deinstitutionalization from state mental hospitals of chronically ill patients is the theme that runs through the modern era of public psychiatry. From 1993 to 2003, several new elements of service appeared at the CMHC, including ACT, homeless outreach, new services for co-occurring mental health and substance-use disorders, and incipient recovery programs and peer services, which would become much more fully developed in the following years. Table 6-2 illustrates these changes. Both ACT and homeless outreach were essential elements of community services development, which characterized the previous period but did not arrive on the scene at the CMHC until after the arbitrary limit this narrative has set for the end of that period. By the end of the period of mainstreaming, the array of services at the CMHC was reasonably complete. Some critical elements remained and were picked up in the next period of development.

With this background, consider the following case example, which illustrates much of the new capacity for care at the CMHC. Robert was a single, homeless 28-year-old man diagnosed with paranoid schizophrenic illness. He was admitted to the hospital for the first time at 21 years of age. He was hospitalized four times subsequently and exhausted his opportunities for living with family or friends because of his disorganized, disruptive, and sometimes antagonistic behavior. He had become homeless and was living in a tent under a bridge at the intersection of two interstates in downtown New Haven. Furthermore,

Table 6-2 Service Type or Benefit by Period in Modern Public Psychiatry

Service Type or Benefit	Post–WW II	CMH	CSS	Main
Asylum, chronic hospitalization	X			
Acute inpatient hospitalization		X	X	X
Nursing home, long-term care		X	X	X
Partial hospitalization, intensive outpatient			X	X
Routine outpatient, ambulatory care		X	X	X
Emergency room	X	X	X	X
Urgent care		X	X	X
Crisis intervention		X	X	X
Neighborhood clinics		X		
Prevention, early intervention		X		
Assertive community treatment				X
Co-occurring services				X
Vocational rehabilitation			X	X
Psychosocial rehabilitation	X		X	X
Case management, community support programs			X	X
Residential services			X	X
System development, local mental health authorities			X	X
Outreach to homeless				X
Recovery, quality of life goals				X
Peer services				X
Integrated primary medical care				
Medicaid Medicare		X	X	X
Supplemental Security Income Social Security Disability Insurance		X	X	X

Abbreviations: CMH, Community Mental Health; CSS, Community Services and Systems; Main, Mainstreaming; Post–WW II, Post–World War II.

through life on the streets, he had begun to dabble in multiple substance use. His most consistent drug of choice was marijuana. His drug use and disorganized behavior on public streets led to his arrest for disorderly conduct. A forensic team member picked him up in a court diversion program and referred him back to a treatment team at the CMHC. He did not attend appointments. After several months the homeless outreach team found him under the bridge, then spent five months winning his confidence in order to convince him to enter a psychosocial rehabilitation program that was part of the community-based service system. An appointment was made for a complete evaluation by a co-occurring disorders team. He appeared, but was again unable to maintain appointments consistently. A referral was made to the ACT team that engaged him on the move on the streets. The ACT team was successful in getting him into a new supported-living apartment to get him off the streets. He was encouraged to attend the psychosocial rehab club and did so periodically. As a result of the clinical and community supports, Robert made a stable adjustment to his new living arrangements. The residential placement became an essential platform for his long-term treatment in the community. He was too disorganized, expressing no interest, to become involved in peer-supported warm lines, work opportunities, or peer-supported services at the CMHC.

Robert's treatment and rehabilitation did not end at this point and continued for many years more. Still, his case illustrates how the new service elements introduced at the CMHC during the period of mainstreaming contributed to the success of engaging him in treatment and helping him adjust to life with a serious mental illness in the community. As recovery services grew at the CMHC, the next period of transformation in public psychiatry would add additional opportunities for people like Robert to live fuller lives as members of the community, pursuing self-identified goals, while the system of services supported his recovery.

CONCLUSION

The period of mainstreaming in public psychiatry at the CMHC was a time driven not only by internal challenges, such as new leadership and the need to cope with constricting resources, but also by national general health and welfare policy, financing strategies, and management initiatives taken in response. It was a time when Medicaid rose as a payer of mental health services. Medicaid and, to a lesser extent, Medicare, as well as other payers, began to drive policy development by means of the services they reimbursed and the latent models they used for reimbursement. Accordingly, in contrast to previous periods of development, state agencies for administering Medicaid played important roles in shaping the public system. Many of the developments during this period reinforced an evolving medical model of care for public psychiatry. This model incorporated into biology and psychology perspectives on the whole population, the social environment, and disability. It was a time when diffusion of the mission and change in character of the target population of public psychiatry accelerated change in orientation away from a narrow, almost exclusive, focus on people with serious mental illness. People with substance-use disorders, with co-occurring mental health and substance-use disorders, and people mandated for treatment or diverted from courts as an alternative to incarceration, not to mention victims of disaster, entered the picture. (The next chapter further examines this issue.) These changes set a stage for the next period of transformation, when the medical care of individuals with serious mental illness would rise to prominence as a central focus.

Mainstreaming of psychiatric services and benefits, which has been a major policy goal of psychiatry for more than two decades, would continue to drive change in psychiatry in the next period of public psychiatry. Strategies to integrate psychiatry and primary care—in order to address the shortened life expectancy of people with serious mental illness—would become a major issue in this period. Also, mainstreaming of psychiatric care is probably the most viable strategy for addressing psychiatric burden of disease in the United States. Undoubtedly, this is true for addressing burden of disease in global mental health practice. It seems inevitable that the combination of mainstreaming, policies to integrated primary care of people with serious mental illness, and public health attempts to reduce burden of psychiatric disease, will bring public psychiatry and medicine even closer going forward.

In 2001, the Bush administration formed the New Freedom Commission to recommend social changes that would enable people with disabilities to live responsible, independent, and productive lives in their communities. A New Freedom Commission on Mental Health was part of this major policy initiative. The report, in 2003, of the Commission on Mental Health was the landmark announcement of the beginning of a new period in public psychiatry, one characterized by policies to transform the mental health system. That contemporary period is the topic of the next chapter.

The Period of Transformation and CMHC, 2003 to the Present

The 2003 report on mental health by the President's New Freedom Commission (NFC) (Figure 7-1) shaped the contemporary period of transformation in modern public psychiatry (President's New Freedom Commission on Mental Health, 2003). While an outgrowth of mainstreaming, the new period had a unique character. The NFC report, building on the 1999 report on mental health by the Surgeon General of the United States Public Health Service, recommended a transformation of the public service system, which it characterized as a "shambles."

Several features of this time justify its designation as a separate, new period in public psychiatry, distinct from the preceding one. In response to growing public health data on the shortened life expectancy of people with serious mental illness, the transformation agenda emphasized the integration of mental health and primary care as a central goal. Emanating from primary care, a policy initiative to establish medical homes for the purpose of organizing care was closely related. Also, the transformation agenda included recovery, person-centered care planning, and consumerism. Transitioning into this new period, the tasks of public psychiatry expanded to include disaster readiness after the terrorist attacks of September 11, 2001. In addition, during the period of transformation, forensic community-based clinical services appeared as a new, specialized service element. The developments associated with this new period continued to diffuse the focus of public psychiatry on people with serious mental illness.

THE DMHAS AND THE CMHC IN 2003

In the state of Connecticut, the recommendations of a 2000 Governor's Blue Ribbon Commission on Mental Health continued to guide policy directions for the Department of Mental Health and Addiction Services (DMHAS; Kirk, 2009). The commission concluded that the mental health system in Connecticut "faced an emerging crisis... that must

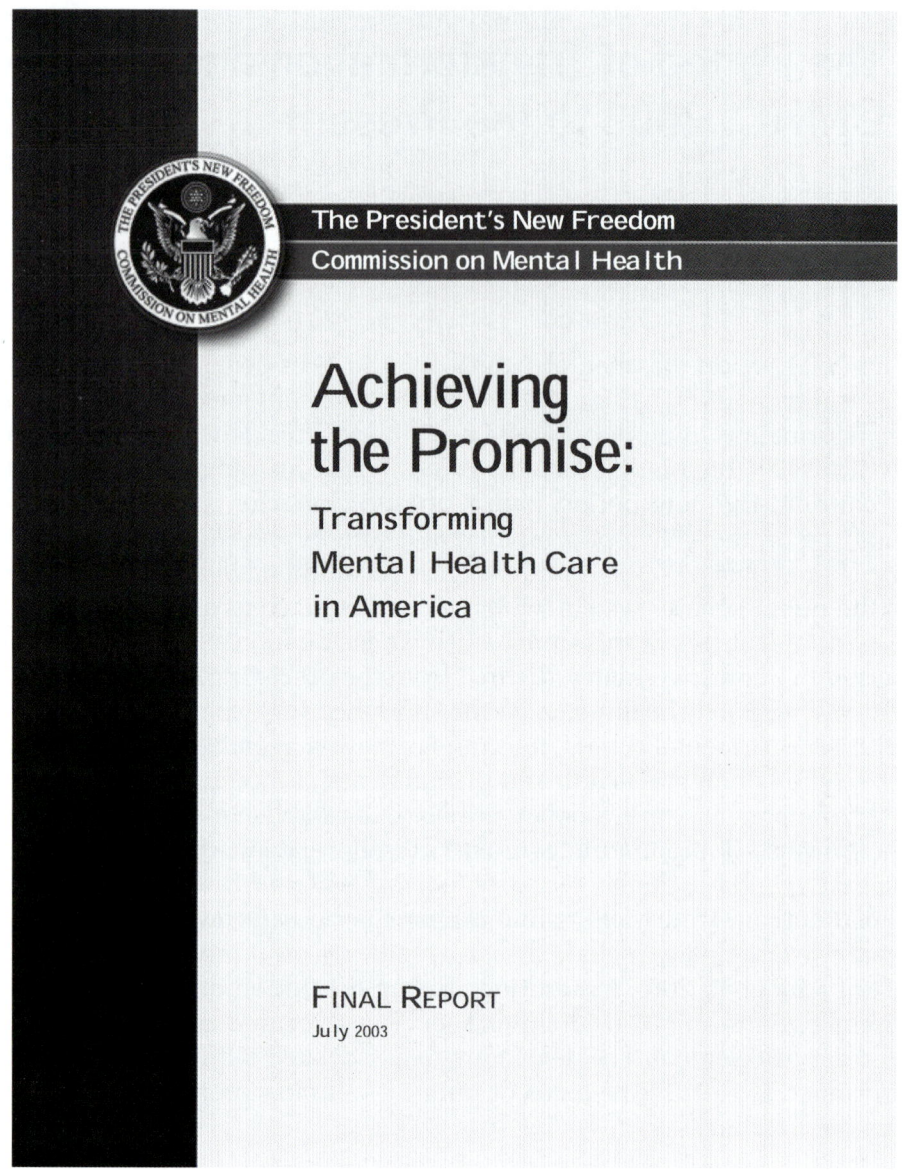

Figure 7-1 Title page of the New Freedom Commission Report of 2003.

be addressed." After the commission report, the DMHAS set a goal to establish itself as a leader among other state mental health authorities in the country, with emphasis on recovery. Grants from the Substance Abuse and Mental Health Services Administration (SAMHSA), as well as state general fund money, financed several initiatives, including attention to comorbidity of mental and substance-use disorders, which unfolded along with a large transformation grant from SAMHSA, built around the theme of recovery.

The Connecticut Mental Health Center (CMHC) and its leadership, though faced with repeated fiscal challenges, were stable on entering the new period of transformation. New service elements appeared, but none constituted a fundamental reorientation or required a pervasive reorganization of the institution. The relationships among the CMHC, the DMHAS, and the Yale Department of Psychiatry (YDP) were steady. The partnership itself, despite minor conflict over a lease agreement related to a planned building addition, was also stable. In short, the CMHC entered the new period on an even keel.

The major events and developments of the period of transformation at the CMHC are summarized in the chronology provided in Table 7-1.

The tone in this chapter, in contrast to earlier ones, evolves into a more conditional and tentative consideration of key variables that are still active and hold consequences for the future of the CMHC, the DMHAS, and the field of public psychiatry in general. It is too early to say with confidence what the outcomes will be. Still, it is important to consider the years since 2003 as a prelude to the discussion in the final chapter of future directions in public psychiatry.

Table 7-1 Chronology at the CMHC of the Period of Transformation, 2003-10

2003	The New Freedom Commission publishes report
2005	R-25 research training grant coalesces academic program on SMI
2005	Public health initiatives at the CMHC
2006	NASMHPD report on shortened life expectancy of people with SMI
2006	Forensic, community-based clinical services
2006	Medicare Part D
2007	AHA report on the acute care crisis in general hospitals
2007	CMHC forensic, community-based clinical services begin
2008	Interim leadership of YDP (Sledge)
2008	Financial and economic crisis in the US
2008	Parity legislation for MH insurance (Medicare and commercial)
2009	Dedication of a building addition for Latino services and preclinical research expansion
2009	New leadership for the CMHC (Sernyak), the YDP (Krystal), and the DMHAS (Rehmer)
2010	Health care reform: the Patient Protection and Affordable Care Act

THE NEW FREEDOM COMMISSION

The 2003 report of the NFC on Mental Health came from the first presidential commission on mental health in a quarter century. It concluded—as had the surgeon general in 1999, the Carter Commission in 1979, and the congressional commission of 1955—that the public mental health system was in trouble. The commission described the system as a "patchwork relic" and declared it was "in shambles," The commission called for "transformation" of the mental health system, rather than incremental change, using recovery as an organizing principle. The NFC completed its report under a presidential admonition not to recommend new federal spending or programs. This policy of the Bush administration reflected a federalist political philosophy that the federal government ought not to be directly involved in solving the problem beyond its role in generating analysis and developing a roadmap for change. Rather, the commission presumed that the solutions would depend on state initiatives, state plans under Medicaid, and enterprising local communities.

The NFC recommended transformation by focusing on six goals:

(1) understanding that mental health is essential to overall health;
(2) making mental health both consumer and family driven;
(3) eliminating disparities in mental health services and outcomes;
(4) accomplishing routine, early mental health screening, assessment, and referral to services;
(5) delivering excellent mental health care through best practices and discoveries from new research; and
(6) using technology to improve access to mental health care through personal health information systems and introduction of electronic medical records (EMRs).

In Connecticut, a seventh goal was added in regard to the need for workforce development. Most of this agenda seemed familiar at the time. Indeed, virtually all the same recommendations were included in the report of the surgeon general of 1999.

It took a few years for the federal government to operationalize the recommendations of the NFC and sponsor demonstration grants in states. In 2005, SAMHSA issued a transformation "road map" and awarded competitive demonstration grants to seven states, including the DMHAS of Connecticut. As part of the new federalism, states had considerable latitude to develop local solutions within the framework created by the NFC goals. Dissemination and implementation of the lessons learned in the demonstrations would depend on local initiative and the fiscal health of the states. Within a few years, the economic recession of 2008 and the dire fiscal condition of the states put a damper on this strategy. Still, transformation remained the major policy guidance for public psychiatry for the next seven years from its appearance in 2003.

Perhaps more important than what the NFC did, such as highlighting the importance of evidence-based practices and interventions in the community, was what it did not do. The report did not recommend a return to the development of a special system of services devoted exclusively to caring for individuals with serious mental illness. In other words, there was no revival of "exceptionalism" exemplified by the periods of community mental health and community services development from 1966 to 1993. Some voices in public psychiatry still advocated for a return to special federal programs in order to meet the needs of seriously ill patients. The NFC did not recommend such a course, consistent with its political mandate not to incur new spending and also with the fundamental policy directions of psychiatry since 1993, subsumed under the concept of mainstreaming (Frank and Glied, 2006).

INTEGRATION OF MENTAL HEALTH AND PRIMARY CARE

Historically, the original community mental health legislation created an expectation that community-based mental health centers would integrate with general hospitals and medical clinics. This did not occur, largely as a function of the absence of specific funding or incentives to achieve integrated care. Low income, uninsured psychiatric patients gravitated to community mental health centers, and those with employer-based insurance found their way to the general hospitals. People with entitlements flowed both ways. During mainstreaming, carved-out financing under independent and often competing managed care contracts and services discouraged collaboration and integration. The assertion of the surgeon general in 1999 that "There is no health without mental health," signaled renewed attention at the policy level on integration of psychiatry and other medical disciplines.

The lead recommendation of the NFC was to establish mental health care as a clinical service central to overall health care. Elimination of carve-outs in both the private and public sectors would become an important strategy for accomplishing the goal of providing prompt and adequate psychiatric evaluation and interventions for patients with primary medical problems. By 2006, there was a growing appreciation that individuals with serious mental illness had severely shortened life expectancy (see below). Hence, conversely, a rationale emerged to integrate mental health with primary care in order to reduce early mortality from chronic diseases such as hypertension, diabetes, and coronary artery disease. These reciprocal processes of integrating mental health and primary care became major building blocks in a transformation policy to mainstream mental health care of people with serious mental illness into primary care.

A state owned and operated facility such as the CMHC could only tackle these major goals with new general fund appropriations, which were virtually impossible to obtain, or with a substantial reallocation of existing resources to solve the problem. In some minds, the latter seemed an inappropriate use of scarce dollars appropriated for mental health care. Accordingly, the CMHC leadership undertook the challenge of integration by considering how to support community health centers and private nonprofit agencies in revenue-based resource and service expansion. The planning for service expansion included two goals. One was collaboration with primary care services to address the shortened life expectancy among those with serious mental illness. A second goal was to expand mental health services and widen the safety net of public psychiatric services in the same agencies by encouraging and support-ing their mental health services. Specifically, the CMHC began to collab-orate more closely with federally qualified health centers because their favorable cost-based reimbursement under Medicaid made expansion possible. This strategy of integration helped solve the problem of insuffi-cient resources at a state owned and operated facility such as the CMHC. It is an ongoing story that will play out over the next several years.

MEDICAL HOMES

By 2008, the concept of patient-centered medical homes emerged in pub-lic mental health discussions. The concept came out of pediatrics and primary care, which had developed it over several years as a fundamen-tal reorganization of medical care in order to better manage chronic dis-eases and reduce medical specialty costs. It was another vehicle for the integration of primary care and mental health.

The prospect of a medical home raised a question about how psychia-trists and other mental health professionals might effectively consult to primary care practices. Though common in general hospitals, consul-tation was rare in public practice in New Haven. The development of medical homes might take psychiatrists at the CMHC outside the clinic walls and engage them with their medical colleagues on medical turf at the community health clinics. Also the prospect of medical homes raised the possibility that community mental health centers, as the principal caregivers for people with serious mental illness, might serve as medical homes for this special population. Both of these possibilities remain unfulfilled, and the prospects for a movement toward medical homes is uncertain.

At the CMHC, the possibility of qualifying as a medical home remained on the horizon as a goal that would require considerable preparation of psychiatrists as well as of the institution itself. It would require the education of public psychiatrists for a new role in screening for common general health problems. For the institution, it would require EMRs. Both tasks, which were related to medical homes, dovetailed into the undertaking of responsibility for improving the shortened life expectancy of people with serious mental illness.

CMHC COLLABORATIONS WITH PRIMARY CARE

In Yale School of Medicine (YSM), beyond the core relationship to the YDP, the CMHC maintained a long-standing collaboration with Yale Primary Care (YPC), a subsection of internal medicine not only at the YSM but also the Yale New Haven Hospital (YNHH). This relationship had been formed many years earlier in faculty collaborations regarding the diagnosis and treatment of alcohol-related disorders. The CMHC formalized the relationship in 1990 with a contract with YPC for primary care consultation at the CMHC. There were two platforms for the relationship. One was the primary care clinic located in, and financed by, the general hospital. The other was the CMHC medical clinic where physicians of YPC saw referrals in consultation. The medical clinic at the CMHC was an early example of co-location of services. Patients could be referred back and forth between the two platforms depending on need, such as subspecialty consultation, and capacity to independently keep appointments.

The 2006 National Association of State Mental Health Program Directors report on the 25-year shorter life expectancy of people with serious mental illness made the CMHC relationship to YPC essential. In 2009 and beyond, YPC and the CMHC collaborated in grant applications to demonstrate co-location of services, building on this long-standing relationship. Furthermore, the CMHC began to systematically build relationships with the two federally qualified health centers in New Haven. There were two potential benefits for the population with serious mental illness served at the CMHC. First, the integration of mental and primary care would better address their general health problems. Second, these collaborations potentially expanded access to mental services at the community health clinics through their own internal mental health services. These services had already expanded in recent years under policies of the Health Services and Resources Agency during the Bush administration. The financially viable mental health services at the community health centers, where reimbursement rates are paid by Medicaid based on the actual cost of care, offered an opportunity not available in the state owned and operated CMHC. The possibility that integrated primary care expanded access to mental health services was a powerful added incentive to move in this direction.

RECOVERY, PERSON-CENTERED CARE, AND PEER SERVICES

The NFC report gave tremendous impetus to recovery as the goal of mental health treatment and support, not only nationally but also at the CMHC. During the period of transformation, the CMHC widely implemented person-centered care, an evidence-based practice that supported the recovery movement. It held fundamental implications for clinical practice. Person-centered care had been under study at the CMHC, funded through a National institute of Mental Health (NIMH) grant. This practice was extended to all the clinical teams of ambulatory services by means of another grant to the DMHAS from the Centers for Medicaid and Medicare Services. The centerwide implementation of person-centered care required orientation and retraining of medical and professional staff throughout the CMHC.

Person-centered care dovetailed into and expanded a broad medical model as a framework for public psychiatry practice. It was necessary to conceptualize a medical model that viewed recipients of care, as well as their families, as active and not passive participants, who would drive the goals and process of care. While this change could be seen as another challenge to professional autonomy and prerogatives, the inherent principle was really time-honored and fundamental to good, responsive care. The trick was continuing to nurture the importance of independent, professional judgment while advocating the value of integrating recovery into a professional model that accommodated an essential participant and point of view.

The expansion of person-centered care reinforced and added vibrancy to the recovery agenda for the CMHC. Person-centered care required a new way of thinking about clinical planning, using language that did not pigeonhole people as a passive recipients with symptoms, for whom clinician-dictated restrictive goals of symptom reduction would suffice. Rather, the person who was ill was an active player who brought goals of living fully and responsibly in the community to the process of treatment planning. It empowered people with mental illnesses to have a greater role in treatment planning and determining the services they would receive. Person-centered care required that patients and their selected representatives would, if necessary, be invited into treatment planning meetings. Instead of people with mental illness trying to fit into the procrustean clinical programs of the treatment team, the person became the hub for mobilizing a variety of services from multiple sources and agencies to meet his or her personal need in an individualized plan of care. The process represented an excellent example of consumer driven care, in contrast to consumer models rooted in commercial experience.

> Person-centered care empowered people with mental illnesses to have a greater role in treatment planning.

Insurance companies and entitlement programs seized on person-centered care as a possible strategy for controlling costs, both in the public and private sectors. Patient-centered care highlighted the role of patients as consumers of services. Payers saw the opportunity and ran with it. For example, in the public sector, some state Medicaid programs began to use the concept of patient-centered care as a strategy for controlling the costs of long-standing, optional services for people with serious mental illnesses. The CMS gave states the opportunity to introduce patient choice into benefit selection, in circumstances where wise selection according to the needs of a chronic illness rather than to simple cost, was far from guaranteed. This change posed a challenge to an implicit and prevailing assumption from the period of community services and system development that mental health system managers or policy makers knew what was best both in system or benefit design.

The period of transformation was also a time when peer services blossomed at the CMHC. Two vehicles account for this development. The Program on Recovery and Community Health at the CMHC obtained a grant to study the roles of peers in primary care. This grant provided training and supervision of peers as "coaches" for psychiatric patients in the emergency room and primary care center of YNHH. This role also extended to the CMHC, where peers served as coaches on the urgent care service and the acute inpatient unit. The peers helped their counterparts, who were more acutely ill, to understand what to expect, fill out screening forms, participate actively in treatment planning, and pass time. Beyond these new roles, a peer steering group (under supervision) staffed an evening, telephone "warm" line for people in crisis. Also, the group managed a small amount of funds to support microeconomic development ideas created by individuals among them.

On an administrative level, the CMHC systematically found advisory positions for peers at all levels of the institution. These advisory roles ranged from specific programs within the recovery program itself to the institutional board and the executive committee of the local mental health authority. Peers also held positions in the DMAS, which was responsible for governance of the institution.

RESEARCH EDUCATION ON SERIOUS MENTAL ILLNESS FOR PSYCHIATRIC RESIDENTS

In 2005, the CMHC, under the leadership of Dr. Bruce Wexler, competed for and won an R-25 training grant from the NIMH for research education on chronic mental illness. The grant supported training of advanced psychiatric residents for academic careers in public psychiatry. The grant application identified many of the CMHC faculty members, who were as yet unaffiliated with research divisions of the YDP, as mentors for the research fellows. The shared teaching responsibility served as a cohesive force in pulling together clinical research on serious and persistent mental illness at the CMHC. The spectrum of research ranged from early intervention for psychosis risk-syndromes to medication effectiveness studies, evaluation of interventions for diabetes and metabolic syndrome to study of wellness programs (Jacobs and Griffith, 2007). The new teaching program reinforced strands of development that began in 1984, when the CMHC instituted its first academic program on serious and persistent mental illness and included the recovery program, which had reinforced the CMHC in its own right in 2000. The grant success was a building block in a process that would ultimately lead to recognition of this critical domain of clinical research as a research division of the YDP. It is an example of how an agenda in public psychiatry helped shape the YDP in a way that gave academic recognition to the needs of people with serious mental illness as well as to an essential professional responsibility of psychiatry.

INTEGRATION OF MENTAL HEALTH AND SUBSTANCE-USE CARE

Though the integration of mental health and substance-use services did not figure in the six major goals of the NFC, it was embedded in the idea of person-centered care, recovery, and the quality goal. A federal action plan, developed by SAMHSA, recommended the integration of these rather separate domains of care for treatment of people with co-occurring disorders. The DMHAS was successful in obtaining a SAM-

HSA demonstration grant for integration of these services. The demonstration grant played into, and reinforced, a long-standing goal of the CMHC to achieve full integration of the entire institution by training all clinicians to be dually competent, at least for the purposes of evaluation. This institutional goal was dictated by the change over time in the patient population, in which co-occurring disorders became the most common presenting clinical problem at the front door. A main obstacle to integration was the task of bringing together clinicians with two distinct clinical cultures. Mental health clinicians had a foundation in psychotherapy and supportive interventions, and substance-use clinicians were rooted more in motivational strategies to engage people in treatment. Motivational interviewing, which was developed for the evaluation of need for addictions treatment, became a useful skill in both camps and helped bridge the gap. Suicidal risk assessment, which was a core clinical skill in both domains, also served to bridge the two.

PUBLIC HEALTH PERSPECTIVES

The NFC heralded psychiatric public health as an important arena for public psychiatry. Public health incorporates prevention; early intervention; health promotion; contingency planning for threats to the public health such as disasters or influenza epidemics; categorical programs for groups at high risk for burden of disease or documented to have disparate clinical outcomes; and public education. Psychiatric public health programs can trace their antecedents back to the community mental health movement of 1963-82, when community practice accorded attention to public health principles of prevention. Prevention, early intervention, and outreach to low income and underserved populations were integral to community mental health programs of that period. The NFC report made it timely and important to return to a focus on public health principles and practice, thereby bringing balance into comprehensive, public, mental health, and addictions programs.

The NFC noted that American society invested inadequately in programs and services at the front end of the trajectory of psychiatric illness. In contrast, enormous resources were committed to tertiary care of disabled individuals with serious mental illnesses and addictions. The NFC report recommended more focus on the early stages of illness. Many of the people falling ill for the first time were at high risk of becoming disabled. Specifically, the NFC report recommended in its fourth goal that mental health screening be improved in order to enable timely clinical assessment (early detection) and referral to continuing services if necessary. The commission intended that screening, in collaboration with primary care, become common practice.

Echoing the recommendations of the NFC, the NIMH published a report in 2006 that characterized the burden of psychiatric disease on the American population as "one of the greatest public health challenges in contemporary medicine" (Insel and Fenton, 2005). This article emphasized that psychiatry in particular faced major public health tasks and created a context for their resolution as part of mainstream medicine. Also, the head of the federal Center for Mental Health Services highlighted the importance in the twenty-first century of public health in public psychiatry (Power, 2009). In her discussion, the administrator described prevention, early intervention, attention to social variables (such as disparities in outcomes for high-risk groups), and a focus not only on disease but also on wellness and resilience. To these might be added programs to address the shortened life expectancy of people with serious mental illness, mortality from suicide, and the introduction of burden of disease metrics into clinical conversation, with an aim to reduce disability for individuals and demands on families.

Arguably, public health data documented, defined, and signaled problems needing correction. The concept of burden of disease and data from the Global Burden of Disease study demonstrated the high ranking of psychiatric disorders among all diseases placed psychiatric disorders squarely on the agenda for state, federal, and international program initiatives (Murray and Lopez, 1996). The Report on Mental Health by the surgeon general, which concluded that the mental health system was in shambles, set the stage for the NFC, which articulated a transformation agenda. A report by National Association of State Mental Health Program Directors (NASMHPD) on a shortened life expectancy for individuals with serious mental illness demanded a response from psychiatry and primary care (NASMHPD, 2006). Large-scale studies by services researchers exposed the false claims of large pharmaceutical companies that were marketing new generations of antipsychotic drugs at very high cost (Lieberman et al., 2005). Finally, public health data on persistently high morbidity rates created the framework for a NIMH report calling for new directions in psychiatric research (Insel, 2009).

PUBLIC HEALTH AT THE CMHC

At the CMHC, prevention programs had been consolidated into a single unit, the Consultation Center, at the time when federal, categorical community mental health funding ended. These programs, under the leadership of Dr. David Snow and colleagues, followed a community consultation and prevention-research agenda on a broad range of topics. They included, among others, prevention of drug abuse in preteens, prevention of domestic violence, and programs targeting high-risk groups such as seniors (Jacobs and Griffith, 2007). The Consultation Center established relationships to epidemiology and services research at the Yale School of Public Health. As a result of these efforts, the Consultation Center became a nationally recognized leader in prevention education. In 2004, the NIMH awarded it a training grant to support prevention-research education for postdoctoral fellows. In this way, through a long fallow period for public health in public psychiatry, the Consultation Center helped to maintain expertise in public health at the CMHC.

This was another example of an academic program sustaining an important stream of public psychiatry that was at risk of withering away because of funding and ideological vicissitudes. When national policy discussions through the NFC returned to the topics of prevention and early intervention, the Consultation Center was an important building block for participation in the transformation agenda. Furthermore, a population perspective on disease and health care intrinsic to public health served to counterbalance a clinical perspective built on single cases. To grasp the mental health of the community, it is essential periodically to step back from case-by-case experience and consider the needs of and services for the whole population.

One of the most important new initiatives at the CMHC was the inception of an early intervention program for first-episode psychosis. Building on the work of Drs. Thomas McGlashan and Scott Woods and their colleagues, which began before the NFC formed and stemmed from innovative studies in Australia, the CMHC developed a new research clinic, Specialized Treatment Early in Psychosis (STEP). STEP mounted special screening and interventions necessary for prompt, efficient intervention in the course of first episodes of psychotic illness. The special program included use of low dose antipsychotic medicines to treat incipient symptoms, engagement in educational and work coaching to prevent the onset of prolonged disability, and active involvement of the family in psychoeducation. The clinic recruited patients successfully from around the state and became a model for early intervention for the DMHAS. The clinical service of the research clinic became a platform for the collection of data and for grant applications to support the demonstration, evaluation, and dissemination of this innovative approach.

Beyond early intervention, a public health perspective helped to address several pressing problems in the delivery of service to the CMHC target population. Perhaps the largest public health challenge of all was the need to improve the life expectancy and reduce the burden of disease among people with serious mental ill-ness. The CMHC began to mobilize resources by recruiting psychiatrists, who were dually boarded, certified in psychia-try and medicine. Also, the institutional leadership oriented faculty staff members

> Perhaps the largest public health challenge was to improve life expectancy and reduce the burden of disease.

to the challenge of increasing life expectancy. Further, as 60–90% of sui-cides are associated with psychiatric illness, a focused approach to sui-cide prevention addressed a major cause of mortality in the target population. A suicide prevention program promised to be particularly important for young adults, whose rates of suicide were the third leading cause of death. In the arena of addictions, a relapse prevention program for tobacco use, establishment of a smoke-free hospital campus, and a gambling prevention program held promise to address current national and local epidemics. In addition, the CMHC began group meetings for high-risk children of parents who suffered from psychotic disorders, in an effort to mitigate the risk of illness as the children grew older. Among the public health challenges was behavioral health-related disaster plan-ning in anticipation of influenza epidemics or man-made disasters. All these were seen as an opportunity to get ahead of the curve with regard to public health programs in responding to the national agenda for trans-formation of the mental health system.

HEALTH CARE DISPARITIES

Stemming from the surgeon general's report and a follow-up publication on health care disparities in mental health, and related to the goals of the NFC report, a major challenge in the early years of the new century was to bring outcomes up to the highest level possible for everyone served at the CMHC. It made sense that cross-cultural competence would help, when connected with a commitment to high quality services. Otherwise, the cultural competence would become a tangential activity and a false promise. Essentially, the CMHC proceeded with the philosophy that the key contribution of cross-cultural competence was to enhance access to, engagement with, and retention in treatment among underserved racial and cultural groups. If the institution could effectively meet and hold anyone in evaluation and treatment, thereby improving access, the clini-cal expertise in various evidence-based treatments would deliver the best outcomes possible.

In order to address these issues, the CMHC built on a long-standing tradition of serving low income people in the community. The institution needed to add to that foundation a refining knowledge of cross-cultural variation. The most focused and substantial development during this period was a series of improvements in the care of monolingual Latinos. Using the strategy of building an educational program for Latino professionals as an academic program under Dr. Luis Anez-Nava and colleagues, the CMHC grew a bilingual, bicultural staff of professionals and mental health workers at its Hispanic Clinic. The academic nature of the programs enhanced an ability to recruit professionals in a perennial buyer's market. Furthermore, the CMHC was successful in convincing local legislators to provide state funds to expand the clinic for New Haven to the surrounding greater metropolitan area. Finally, with the construction of a building addition to the CMHC, an opportunity developed to bring in these services from a satellite location and integrate them into the main building and programs.

By the conclusion of this period, the Latino services at the CMHC led the state in demonstrating an approach to cross-culturally competent services for a particular ethnic group. It was the addition of cross-cultural and social competence to biological and psychological approaches to treatment that made this clinic a quintessential program of its kind in public psychiatry.

FORENSIC, COMMUNITY-BASED CLINICAL SERVICES

While multiple developments were unfolding, largely subsumed under the rubric of transformation, the agenda for public psychiatry at the CMHC expanded. Beginning in 2006, in response to the interest of a local state assemblyman Representative William Dyson, who found pilot money for a demonstration project, the CMHC began special clinical services for people leaving prison on parole or probation. In 2009, a horrifying incident of home invasion and multiple murders by parolees in Cheshire, Connecticut, prompted a governor's commission and parole reform. This incident also underscored a critical need for community-based forensic clinical services. Adding to existing alternatives to incarceration programs, which were linked to drug courts, the net impact was the creation of a substantial nucleus of clinical services specifically associated with forensic populations. This critical mass required more attention, coordination, and management. Many of the new population were substance users, and all faced fundamental problems in reintegrating into the community. The problem of reintegration was aggravated by loss of driver's licenses at the time of incarceration. Parolees had no satisfactory form of identification in order to access basic housing and other social services. Further, there was the challenge of coordinating clinical services with court-based community monitoring, which had little or no clinical knowledge, experience, or judgment. For the purpose of addressing all these challenges the CMHC organized a new division of community-based forensic clinical services with an administrative head. The pilot project in 2006 led to generalized funding for such programs throughout the state. These programs will grow under the federal Second Chance Act of 2008, which will provide federal support for such services.

YOUNG, CHRONICALLY ILL ADULTS

Additionally, the CMHC was engaged in developing special clinical programs for young adults who were leaving institutional placements of the Connecticut Department of Children and Families (DCF). Another horrifying incident in 2008, which involved the murder of a mentally ill teenager by her mentally ill peers in Hartford, placed renewed emphasis on the need for young adult services. These services were especially important for 18-year-olds, who were aging out of the programs of the state Department of Children and Family Services. These chronically ill and often chronically institutionalized young adults had many challenging problems. They essentially required special residential placements, supported by an assertive community treatment team of interdisciplinary clinicians. Again, the CMHC organized a special clinical program to meet the needs of this population. These new services built on a small clinic for children in the town of West Haven, which was a vestige of the community mental health period when federal policy required special child services. As the institution began to gain experience, the clinic recognized a frequent presentation of psychosexual problems in these young adults. This clinical demand set an agenda for professional education, which featured as one performance improvement goal in 2007. All the clinical faculty and staff of the CMHC thereby acquired a new set of skills not previously, or at least not recently, a part of their clinical portfolio.

MISSION OF THE CMHC

At the CMHC and the DMHAS, both the periods of mainstreaming and transformation were associated with a change in character of target population and expansion of the range of clinical services away from the singular goal of serving individuals with serious mental illness, which had dominated the community services and system development period of public psychiatry. Since then, categorical funding of services for several special target groups had grown substantially in order to solve social and clinical problems. The special groups included homeless mentally ill people with co-occurring mental health and substance-use disorders; mentally ill people being diverted from incarceration; people transitioning out of prison; and young adults. The net result was substantial evolution in the presenting problems of people, who applied for treatment at the CMHC. No longer was it mainly individuals with serious mental illness (practically the exclusive focus of the previous decade), but also people with co-occurring disorders, forensic cases, homeless mentally ill, and chronically ill young adults with unique needs. It is true that many of the special groups described above meet a definition of serious and persistent mental illness, but not all do so. It is the latter that account for the change in mission

As a result of the changes described here, it became practically impossible to define the target population, despite many attempts in state agency meetings to do so. Rather, the more sensible exercise was to itemize the populations served, set priorities, and then try to achieve a balanced set of services. A central conviction for the CMHC in the face of target population diffusion was to sustain a core commitment to serving people with serious mental illness in the circumstances of competing demands and constricting resources. The CMHC accomplished this goal largely through the development of special programs for this population. These include the initiation of early intervention in first-episode psychosis program; development of programs for high-risk groups such as teenagers and young adults; a rededication to achieving dual competency to treat co-occurring mental health and substance-use disorders in this population; a commitment to recovery programs; renewed efforts to integrate treatment and rehabilitation services; and a growing commitment to the co-location within community mental health centers of behavioral and primary care, using disease management and wellness programs. Innovative relationships to federally qualified community health centers and grant funding facilitated these goals. Continuing attention to these goals and to new opportunities as they arise can help to sustain services for individuals with serious and persistent mental illness.

MEDICARE PART D

Before the health care reform of 2010, the single most important federal initiative in financing of health care during the period of transformation occurred in 2006 with the enactment and implementation of Medicare Part D. It was a momentous change in financing of pharmaceutical treatment under Medicare. At the CMHC, the largest impact occurred for low income patients who were dually eligible for Medicare and Medicaid. Local and state programs for financing medications were replaced by the new federal entitlement. Medicare Part D established competing pharmacy benefit plans that implemented utilization management to control costs. For the most part, this change did not disrupt treatment of patients, though it did require more attention by clinicians to the various formularies of the drug plans and the annual enrollment process for patients. After considerable preparation and education, both for prescribers and patients, the changes went smoothly in Connecticut at the CMHC. As an alternative to local and state plans, Medicare Part D was an example of an expanded, mainstream federal entitlement that benefited people with serious mental illness.

CRISIS IN ACUTE CARE

Among the special reports available on the website of the NFC was one on a growing crisis in acute care services (President's New Freedom Commission, 2003). It was not included in the final published report. The crisis encompassed inpatient beds and crisis-respite beds. In Connecticut, following a 2007 American Hospital Association report on solutions to this crisis, the issue peaked and resulted in a governor's commission (American Hospital Association, 2007; Governor's Hospital System Strategic Task Force Report, 2008) that focused on gridlock, both in the emergency rooms and on inpatient units of general hospitals. Fiscal crises in most Connecticut hospitals, including two threatened with insolvency, composed the background for the public discussion. In 2008, the commission made several recommendations to improve reimbursement and reduce gridlock on general hospital units by improving lower levels of service for patients from hospital units and diversion of patients from emergency rooms into urgent care and crisis or respite services.

In New Haven, responding to an initiative of the largest general hospital, the CMHC began meetings with the hospital vice president in charge of psychiatric services and the psychiatry chief of service. The meetings addressed gridlock in the emergency rooms and on hospital units of the two main general hospitals in the area, where long stays resulted from lack of adequate step-down options. The chief operating officer and chief financial officer of the DMHAS joined the meetings. The local meetings evolved into an exploratory local management project for DMHAS. Documentation of the problem by collecting utilization data led to a Request for Information (RFI) issued by the DMHAS, intended to reorganize services. The reorganization under consideration aimed to divert patients from emergency rooms and from admission to the hospital, and to facilitate discharges. A series of local meetings began to reset the priorities of the mental health managed-service system of the CMHC in order to relieve gridlock, both in the ER and on inpatient units.

The development of this agenda is another example of mainstreaming of public mental health services through integration with general hospital psychiatry. As a final note, the DMHAS at last abandoned its intent to issue a Request for Proposals that would be built on information obtained from responses to the RFI. In part, the interest of the DMHAS flagged as a result of political controversy among private non-profit, mental health providers who feared the initiative might lead to reallocation of resources away from their facilities. The process of joint planning established useful joint efforts by the general hospitals of New Haven and the CMHC to relieve the acute care crisis. Nevertheless, it is quite likely the crisis will continue to play out in the future.

DEINSTITUTIONALIZATION OF NURSING HOMES

Over the modern era of public psychiatry, state hospitals discharged many people with serious mental illness into nursing homes. If they qualified for Medicaid, the entitlement paid the nursing home costs. Though it may have been intended as a step-down level of care from the hospital, for many people the nursing home turned into a permanent living arrangement and a source of long-term care. This process was called trans-institutionalization.

> For many people, the nursing home turned into a permanent living arrangement.

During the period of transformation in Connecticut, nursing homes were faced with persistent budget problems. Many of them had a census of mentally ill patients, which exceeded 50%. Under Medicaid, they were de facto "institutions for mental diseases" (IMD) and as such were at risk of losing Medicaid reimbursement as a function of the Medicaid IMD exclusion of Medicaid. The IMD exclusion was part of the Medicaid legislation to control federal expenditures and hold states responsible for their traditional role in providing hospital care to people with chronic mental illness. To solve this problem, it was necessary to transition stable, chronically ill psychiatric patients from the nursing homes into community-based services.

The DMHAS established a team to survey nursing home residents, identify those suitable for discharge into the community, and arrange community placements with clinical and other support services. The state also developed and obtained approval from the federal government for a Home and Community-Based Services–1915 (c) Waiver that permitted Medicaid to fund community care for people being diverted or discharged from nursing homes. Additionally, the state took part in a Money Follows the Person (MFP) demonstration project through Medicaid intended to rebalance the system as well as cut federal costs. The rationale of the program was to increase the use of less expensive and less restrictive home and community-based, rather than institutional, long-term care services. Flexible use of Medicaid reimbursement and an increase in the federal matching assistance percentage (FMAPP) for 12 months enabled these objectives. States were required to increase their capacity for home and community-based, long-term care and services. Community mental health centers, including the CMHC, augmented by a designated nursing staff position to implement the transition, were instrumental in supporting this project. It was a harbinger of reform of chronic care for people with serious mental illness in nursing homes under the health care reform of 2010.

This initiative represented a special contemporary wave of deinstitutionalization. It was a final stage of deinstitutionalization after the transfer of many patients with serious and persistent mental illness from state hospitals into nursing homes enabled by Medicaid. Finally, deinstitutionalization, the underlying theme of modern public psychiatry, was winding down.

HOUSING FIRST

"Housing first" was an approach to residential services developed by Pathways to Housing in New York City. This program required a reorganization and reorientation of residential services at the CMHC. Most of the residential services at the CMHC were predicated on the idea of services first, which demanded considerable clinical resources that may not have been wanted by the recipient of care. Furthermore, the "housing first" experience provided evidence that clinical services sometimes were not needed in order to reduce readmissions, incarceration, and achievement of stable housing arrangements by the people benefiting from a place to live. This new practice promised to reorient the substantial existing housing resources at the CMHC as well as make more efficient use of clinical resources.

The implications of "housing first" for the identity of the CMHC, if pondered, had a Copernican quality. While the change in identity evolved slowly and progressively, this experience cemented it. The essential problem addressed by "housing first" was the social blight of homelessness, not symptoms of mental illness. Clinicians at the CMHC tended to view the task of finding residential placement for patients as adjunctive. The opposite proved true for many people with serious mental illness with respect to certain outcomes. It is not "clinical services first," but rather "housing first." Housing in some cases was just as potent an intervention as the use of antipsychotic drugs. The CMHC, by extending its services into the community and addressing the needs of patients in recovery who were living in the community, had come a long way in 20 years. The CMHC was no longer the center of the universe, which (though an exaggeration) is not far from how it conceived itself when it first went for accreditation in 1984. At that point, CMHC saw itself as an academic hospital and clinic engaged in traditional biomedical and psychotherapeutic treatments (see chapter 5).

These comments on "housing first" also illustrate an essential dimension of practice in public psychiatry. Public psychiatry must encompass social variables in order to understand mental illness in the community and to implement social interventions in order to be effective. A narrow biomedical approach to care of people with serious mental illness in the community does not get the job done. This realization is inevitable in day-to-day encounters with patients in the community. The "housing first" experience crystallized the issue again for the CMHC.

TRANSLATION

Both person-centered care and "housing first" are examples of evidence-based practice implemented in a timely fashion at the CMHC during the period of transformation. In this way, the institution renewed its efforts to be in the forefront of translation, a term that denotes the transfer of new knowledge from scientific discovery into clinical practice. The report of the NFC emphasized the need, value, and importance of evidence-based treatment. Four years earlier, in 1999, the report of the surgeon general made the same case and placed translation on the agenda of the CMHC, consistent with its identity as an academic institution. In response to these stimuli, the leadership of the CMHC began an annual review of internal academic programs and of the national research literature to identify candidate interventions for translation and implementation. Another example, in addition to those above, was a computer-based, cognitive enhancement intervention to improve work performance of people with serious mental illness and cognitive disability. These interventions were incorporated into strategic plans and performance improvement goals for subsequent years. In this way, the CMHC tried to deliver on the potential and promise of an academic community mental health center.

Chapter 2 argued that translation was not as important a driver of change in contemporary public psychiatry as mainstreaming and transformation. Others might disagree with this point of view (Drake et al., 2003). Given the 17-year lag in the implementation of discovery, scientific evidence and efficient translation (whether a primary or secondary factors in the end) are essential to the evolution of contemporary psychiatry both in the public and private domains.

ELECTRONIC MEDICAL RECORDS

Repeatedly over the past several years the medical staff of the CMHC initiated discussions regarding the development of an EMR. At first, the focus was on computerized physician-ordering systems, in part to reduce errors within a comprehensive patient safety program stimulated by the new quality agenda. In this instance, and in all subsequent EMR initiatives at the CMHC, progress bogged down in discussions with the DMHAS. First, the DMHAS promised to procure a computerized physician-order entry system via statewide bidding. Nothing materialized over the next few years. Later, the DMHAS decided to invest in a recovery-oriented EMR being developed by a computer savvy psychiatrist on its staff who had implemented a Windows-based system at a DMHAS facility. Eventually this project bogged down in the challenge of taking the system from desktop programming in Microsoft to a statewide Web-based system. The time and costs of transferring programs from the laptop to the Web were prohibitive. The recession of 2008 seemed to be a final straw for this project.

In the meantime, many medical staff members at the CMHC had experience in using the EMR of the West Haven Veteran's Medical Center. This system, which is over 30 years old, highly evolved, and easily modifiable for local needs, is free for use to the public. Still, it required a modest budget and resources for maintenance of the system. The resource needs exceeded the capacity of the small information technology unit of the CMHC. The medical staff of the CMHC developed a proposal for the DMHAS to let the facility proceed with adoption of the Veteran's Administration system. Such a plan, and the small investment involved, would serve as an alternative for the DMHAS in the event its in-house project ground to a halt. Repeated frustration with the state bureaucracy, unfortunately, was the recurring history of this project. This initiative by CMHC medical staff was shelved at a time when the commissioner was about to retire and remains undone. Still, it represents an important direction for the CMHC to pursue as it moves forward with multiple aspects of its transformation agenda, such as integrated primary care, qualification as a medical home, and evaluation of efforts to reduce health care disparities, among others.

THE FINANCIAL CRASH AND ECONOMIC RECESSION OF 2008

During the period of transformation, the CMHC continuously coped with a series of fiscal problems caused by the slow recovery of states from the economic recession of 2000-2001. The financial and economic recession of 2008 posed the largest crisis of all. It cut into state revenues and created severe budget deficits for fiscal years 2009 and 2010. As a function of a strong, supportive, and reciprocal relationship with the DMHAS, the CMHC aggressively demonstrated its willingness and ability to implement budget cuts to help the state agency balance its budget. State personnel were cut by 10% and the faculty contract absorbed a $400,000 cutback in the first year. At the same time, the CMHC had to defend the faculty contract that supported medical staff members from targeted cuts of $2 million proposed by the governor's budget director. The CMHC developed a legislative strategy for the latter cut, doing so in concert with the DMHAS, which agreed to make up gaps in the final budget passed by the legislature, which might compromise medical staff services. In short, through the actions of the local legislative delegation, the CMHC avoided the targeted cut of the state budget office and prevented damage to its medical services.

DEDICATION OF A BUILDING ADDITION IN 2009

The dedication of a building addition to the CMHC on January 23, 2009, offered an opportunity to celebrate and renew the partnership between the State of Connecticut and Yale University. The CMHC took the initial step toward a building addition in 1998 (see chapter 6). In the long time between start to finish, the administration of the CMHC surmounted multiple obstacles to its completion. The dedication, attended by the lieutenant governor, the president of Yale University, the mayor of New Haven, the commissioner of the DMHAS, and the legislators who made the addition possible, was a celebration of a 43-year-old partnership that enables the three missions of services, education, and research at the CMHC.

NEW LEADERSHIP AT DMHAS, THE YDP, AND THE CMHC

In July 2009, Dr. John Krystal was appointed chairman of the YDP. At the same time, Dr. Michael Sernyak was appointed director of the CMHC. In October 2009, Ms. Pat Rehmer was appointed commissioner of the DMHAS. Brief vignettes about each of these new leaders are provided in chapter 2. The important point here is that the CMHC and the partnership between the YDP and the DMHAS were entering an entirely new phase of leadership. All three new leaders started in the middle of a health care reform debate in the United States. After the start of the new year, Congress enacted the Patient Protection and Affordable Care (PPAC) Act of 2010. Major change in the financing of mental health care was already afoot by this time.

PARITY LEGISLATION AND HEALTH CARE REFORM

In 2008, Congress passed the Wellstone-Dominici Mental health Parity Act (Figure 7-2), with regard to commercial insurance, and the Medicare Improvements for Patients and Providers Act, which legislated nondiscriminatory mental health insurance benefits under Medicare. Policy and political battles still lie ahead as implementation proceeds. For example, managed care companies have mounted legal challenges because the legislation restricts their traditional strategies for controlling mental health costs. And the extension of parity to Medicaid behavioral managed care is not clear under these acts at this time. Mental health advocates are striving to assure that such plans are included in the regulations being drafted to implement the bill. Nevertheless, nondiscriminatory health insurance for psychiatric disorders was a landmark.

In 2010, Congress enacted, and on March 23 President Obama signed into law, the PPAC Act. It was a national milestone achieved after almost

---

H. R. 1424—117

Subtitle B—Paul Wellstone and Pete Domenici Mental Health Parity and Addiction Equity Act of 2008

SEC. 511. SHORT TITLE.

This subtitle may be cited as the "Paul Wellstone and Pete Domenici Mental Health Parity and Addiction Equity Act of 2008".

SEC. 512. MENTAL HEALTH PARITY.

(a) AMENDMENTS TO ERISA.—Section 712 of the Employee Retirement Income Security Act of 1974 (29 U.S.C. 1185a) is amended—

Figure 7-2 Title page of the Mental Health Parity Act of 2008.

100 years of failed efforts to pass health care reform in the United States. The legislation was massive; some have estimated that implementation of PPHA will generate 30 million pages of regulations. The PPAC Act reformed health care through basic changes in private health insurance policies and Medicaid (National Council for Community Behavioral Health, 2010a and 2010b; Kaiser Family foundation, 2010b). As a critical consideration, Congress included parity for insurance coverage of behavioral disorders. Therefore, the PPAC Act not only extended health care insurance to many uninsured people, but it did so with nondiscriminatory mental health and substance-use benefits. These policy achievements in the course of two years were the holy grail of psychiatric advocates for at least 17 years.

> Three themes dominated discussions on the PPAC Act: access, cost, and quality.

Three themes dominated public discussion in the prelude to passage of the legislation. They were access, cost, and quality. The bill portended major change in all three areas for medicine and psychiatry, including the public sector. The timeline for implementation of health care reform stretches nine years ahead (Kaiser Family Foundation, 2010a). Given concerns about cost, it is likely that Congress will revisit the legislation and significantly modify it over that period. Therefore, at this point in time, it is only possible to speculate where the legislation will lead.

Elements of health care reform under the PPAC Act reinforce basic directions of development from the period of transformation in public psychiatry. These include: integrated primary care; person-centered care; recovery; early intervention and wellness; quality improvement; and introduction of medical information technology. Mainstreaming of behavioral health care into general medical and welfare benefits continues unabated, if not with greater force than before. Thus, it is possible to see the implications of health care reform as an extension of mainstreaming and transformation in public psychiatry.

But, rather than a report of desiderata in mental health care from a commission of professionals and policy makers, the momentous and monumental PPAC Act is a powerful, federal government intervention in how medical services are organized and paid for. The insurance reform and changes in Medicaid under PPAC have the potential to shape practice in medicine, psychiatry, and the public sector for years. The reorganization of chronic care for people with serious mental illness now in nursing homes is a new direction with enormous power to change public psychiatry. Given the scope, nature, and power of health care reform under the PPAC Act, and assuming it is in large part implemented over the years, it seems more reasonable to say that a new period of public psychiatry is opening. Indeed, it may be revolutionary. Public psychiatry will not be the same a decade from now (NCCBH, 2010a).

Public psychiatrists must accept all the implications of this achievement: not only the parity but also the accountability and the quality improvement that goes along with it. They must do so for the purpose of improving access to mental health and substance-use services for the public they serve as professionals. The next, and final, chapter considers the implications of health care reform and other variables shaping the future for public psychiatry, for services to people with serious mental illness, for state departments of mental health, and for community mental health centers, including the state owned and operated CMHC.

SERVICE DEVELOPMENT FOR PEOPLE WITH SERIOUS MENTAL ILLNESS DURING THE PERIOD OF TRANSFORMATION

This chapter concludes with consideration of the service developments at the CMHC, which supported the process of deinstitutionalization and treatment of people with serious mental illness in the community. Among the key additions to the spectrum of available services was integrated primary care, the fundamental new dimension of care for people with serious mental illness. Also, early intervention programs, as well as other public health initiatives (a return of services offered during community mental health), provided a strong strategy for reducing burden of disease. Finally, growth in person-centered care and services led by peers, which blossomed and expanded in this period, deserve mention.

The example of Barbara, an 18-year-old single teenager, who developed difficulty adjusting to her first year at college illustrates these changes. On Barbara's return home from college, her parents noted that she reported bizarre perceptual experiences, interpreted her experience in a paranoid way, and showed no interest in renewing social ties with old friends. The evaluating CMHC clinician believed she was suffering from an incipient psychosis. While in the waiting room of the urgent care service, she was assisted by a peer counselor who helped her fill out the self-reported history and explained what to expect during the evaluation. She was referred to the STEP program, which offered special services for such individuals and their families. She began taking low doses of olanzapine, an antipsychotic medicine. She also underwent a complete assessment of her educational and career aspirations. She was encouraged and supported in resuming study in a few courses at a community college while living at home. Her family participated in multifamily group psychoeducation meetings to learn about their daughter's illness and how they might cope with it effectively. The following September, Barbara made a renewed attempt to attend college where she had started the year before. To support her, a referral was made to the university mental health service. She was in a position to be one of the 20% of people who experience one episode of psychosis and have no recurrence. Barbara's treatment did not end at this point. It already illustrates a few of the new elements of service introduced in this period of transformation.

Another case example illustrates the benefits of integrated primary care. Frank was a 42-year-old divorced man with severe, recurrent schizoaffective illness. Over the years, his clinicians hospitalized him many times. He was followed by one of the outpatient teams at the CMHC, where he was treated with antipsychotics and antidepressants. He no longer worked steadily and led a sedentary life in a single room at a boarding house. In part, as a side effect of earlier treatment with olanzapine, he was obese and had metabolic syndrome. Metabolic syndrome is a group of risk factors for coronary artery disease and adult-onset diabetes mellitus. In addition to obesity, the risk factors include high blood pressure, high fasting blood sugar, and high cholesterol. His clinicians encouraged him to join a weight reduction study where he was supported in following a healthy, low calorie diet. In addition, he routinely exercised in a wellness group. Over nine months, he lost 53 pounds, and his risk factors showed improvement. He felt better physically. He also felt more in control of his life. His appearance improved. He was invited to become a coach in the wellness group. He became energized enough to begin regular attendance at a psychosocial rehabilitation program in the community.

As Table 7-2 indicates, the accrual of services over the years since 1963 created a broad spectrum from which to draw for the purpose of caring for people with serious mental illness. No single period had it all right. All the services were important to practically everyone at some point in the course of a severe and persistent mental illness. It is the accumulated array of services and benefits that lead to the conclusion that, over the past 50 years, people with serious mental illness were "better but not well," in terms of American society meeting their needs for care in the community (Frank and Glied, 2006). It is the accumulation of services that is necessary and must be maintained. This is a big order for a public system that lurches from agenda to agenda and is constrained by budget stringency. This realization places the maintenance of services for people with serious mental illness at the top of priorities in public psychiatry going forward.

Table 7-2 Service Type or Benefit by Period in Modern Public Psychiatry

Service Type or benefit	Post–WW II	CMH	CSS	Main	Trans
Asylum, chronic hospitalization	X				
Acute inpatient hospitalization		X	X	X	X
Nursing home, long-term care		X	X	X	X
Partial hospitalization, intensive outpatient			X	X	X
Routine outpatient, ambulatory care		X	X	X	X
Emergency room	X	X	X	X	X
Urgent care		X	X	X	X
Crisis intervention		X	X	X	X
Neighborhood clinics		X			
Prevention, early intervention		X			X
Assertive community treatment			X	X	X
Co-occurring services				X	X
Vocational rehabilitation			X	X	X
Psychosocial rehabilitation	X		X	X	X
Case management, community support programs			X	X	X
Residential services			X	X	X
System development, local mental health authorities			X	X	X
Outreach to homeless				X	X
Recovery, quality of life goals				X	X
Peer services				X	X
Integrated primary medical care					X
Medicaid Medicare		X	X	X	X
Supplemental Security Income Social Security Disability Insurance		X	X	X	X

Abbreviations: CMH, Community Mental Health; CSS, Community Services and Systems; Main, Mainstreaming; Post–WW II, Post–World War II; Trans, Transformation.

CONCLUSION

Consideration of the recent history of the CMHC in light of the conclusions and goals of the NFC seems to justify the idea of a new contemporary period in public psychiatry, which supplanted mainstreaming.

The only reason to question this judgment is that the current period can also be seen as an extension of mainstreaming, which culminated in the passage of parity legislation and health care reform. Still, the power of a presidential commission and the agenda it set, deserves emphasis, at least for the years immediately following the publication of its recommendations.

By 2010, political and policy changes were piling up one upon another, starting with mainstreaming, then transformation, then parity and health care reform, which can be seen as the culmination of mainstreaming policy goals. On one hand, NFC was recommending transformation of a system it found in disarray. The NFC criticized public psychiatry for going too far in its focus on persistent illness and disability and losing sight of the complete trajectory of behavioral illness, from prevention and acute illness to relapse, chronic illness, and often recovery. True to the federalist philosophy behind it, the NFC recommended local and state initiatives to transform the public sector of services and highlighted the two themes: integration of behavioral health into general health care and recovery.

On the other hand, the logic of mainstreaming was not geared particularly to maintenance of the special spectrum of clinical, rehabilitative, and support services needed by many people with serious mental illness and administered by state mental health authorities. Mainstreaming, in the instance of Medicaid, was a source of support for the special services required by people with serious mental illness. In other instances, such as Medicare and commercial insurance, the process of mainstreaming did not address the special needs of people with serious and persistent mental illness. In order to work well for people with serious mental illness, the process of mainstreaming, which was reinforced powerfully by parity legislation in 2008 and health care reform in 2010, would require a resetting of the long-standing, cost-shifting conflict between state and federal governments as they seek to manage their costs. State and federal governments, as well as the multiple agencies within each level of government, would need to work out new, complementary, and cooperative roles over time.

The circumstances in 2010 suggested that the CMHC was entering a period of rapid, if not revolutionary, change. Indeed, this was true for the whole field of public psychiatry. As public psychiatry faced the future, the best of the times was the promise of expanded access to mental health care for many people, improvements in quality of care, and excitement about discoveries regarding the nature and treatment of psychiatric disorders that lie ahead. For most mental health facilities and clinicians on the ground, the worst of the times portended intensified managed care and cost control, augmented requirements to document and account for service, and the always time-consuming, costly adoption of new technologies, such as the EMR.

At the CMHC, the professional charge was to meet the challenges ahead, while practicing, evaluating, and teaching about them, on behalf of the people the institution serves—in particular, people with severe and persistent mental illness. The final chapter develops an overview of contemporary public psychiatry, reviews the variables that are shaping the future, and offers ideas about future directions at the CMHC and for the field.

Future Directions in Public Psychiatry

> "It was the best of times, it was the worst of times...."
> Charles Dickens, *A Tale of Two Cities*

By 2010, the field of modern public psychiatry had come a long way since the community mental health movement launched in 1963. Deinstitutionalization was an undercurrent throughout this modern era. All of the modern era can be seen as a progressive development of community-based services and supports for people who either were being discharged from state hospitals after long stays or for people who fell ill with a serious mental illness and were at risk of chronic institutionalization.

Development of policy in modern public psychiatry was neither smooth nor consistent. Development of services unfolded by action, reaction, and course correction. The evolution of modern public psychiatry can be seen as a dialectical process, insofar as there is evidence of synthesis or some progress over the years. For example, in reaction to the deplorable conditions of state hospitals in the post–World War II period, the federally funded community mental health movement stimulated the creation of many new community facilities and services. During the period of community services and system development, state mental health authorities regained program development initiative with a focus on chronically ill people, which the previous period had not served well. In addition, emphasis shifted from facility-based services to community-based services. Mainstreaming of health and welfare benefits supervened in part as a function of the fact that evaluations demonstrated that systems offered little or no value for individuals with serious mental illness. Also, 10 years after the opening of the period of mainstreaming, a national presidential commission criticized the public mental health system for an oversized investment in chronic care and disability benefits, while losing sight of early interventions for the purpose of prospectively reducing burden of disease. Further, under managed care, an acute care crisis in mental health developed as a result of the under-reimbursement and closure of psychiatric beds in general hospitals. As a result, because there were not enough beds, it was difficult to hospitalize for acute care as well as, in some cases to, refer for long-term hospitalization in order to best serve clinical and patient needs. Ironically, the modern era had opened with concerns about how to help people get out of hospitals; the contemporary concern was how to get them in, if they needed it.

Over the modern era of public psychiatry at the CMHC, an impressive array of services evolved for people with serious mental illness. By the time health care was enacted in 2010, many questions existed. Was there progress or synthesis, or were modern developments just a series of additions to the hodgepodge? Did the psychiatric public sector of services have a useful and accessible array of special services that had grown over time for people with serious mental illness, or was it in disarray? Was the spectrum of services secure, or was it in jeopardy? Would mainstreaming efforts provide reimbursement for the full spectrum of services needed by people with serious mental illness or not? Over the modern period, were people with serious mental illness "better but not well" (Frank and Glied, 2006), or were they at risk of losing important benefits needed for their care—a function in part of mainstreaming changes and in part of the change in character of the target population in a public system with finite resources. What were the implications of the contemporary scene in public psychiatry for the future of care for people with serious mental illness? This chapter considers these questions and offers ideas about future directions.

A TIME OF CHANGE IN PUBLIC PSYCHIATRY

In 2010, major change was afoot in public psychiatry. The field was midstream in a period of transformation stemming from the 2003 New Freedom Commission (NFC). Local and state initiatives to transform public psychiatry continued to unfold, guided by the goals of NFC and the road map of the Substance Abuse Mental Health Services Administration (SAMHSA). Then, on top of the transformation agenda, President Obama signed into law the Patient Protection and Affordable Care (PPAC) Act of 2010, which has the potential to overtake the transformation agenda by introducing powerful new measures to expand access to psychiatric services through extension of psychiatric benefits at parity to 32 million uninsured people (Figure 8-1). Indeed, a new period of health care reform in public psychiatry seemed to be opening ahead. The next nine-year period, which is the implementation timetable of the new federal legislation, promises to be a period of unprecedented and growing demand for services. Accountability and emphasis on quality go

PUBLIC LAW 111–148—MAR. 23, 2010   124 STAT. 119

Public Law 111–148
111th Congress

An Act

Entitled The Patient Protection and Affordable Care Act.

Be it enacted by the Senate and House of Representatives of the United States of America in Congress assembled,

SECTION 1. SHORT TITLE; TABLE OF CONTENTS.

(a) SHORT TITLE.—This Act may be cited as the "Patient Protection and Affordable Care Act".

(b) TABLE OF CONTENTS.—The table of contents of this Act is as follows:

Mar. 23, 2010
[H.R. 3590]

Patient
Protection and
Affordable Care
Act.
42 USC 18001
note.

Figure 8-1 Title page of The Patient Protection and Affordable Care Act of March 23, 2010.

hand-in-hand with the expanded access in order to control costs. Taken together, all the impending changes may revolutionize health care in the United States. In these circumstances, it is timely to consider emerging trends in public psychiatry, weigh them, and offer ideas about future directions for the field and for the CMHC.

A CONTEMPORARY PROFILE OF PUBLIC PSYCHIATRY

The present picture of public psychiatry is mixed, as it was in 2003 on publication of the *Community Mental Health Journal* issue honoring the fortieth anniversary of the community mental health movement (*Community Mental Health Journal*, 2003). The articles in this special issue reflected both optimistic and pessimistic attitudes about the future. At present, it is hard to know whether to be optimistic or pessimistic about the future.

Beyond optimism and pessimism, in a time of change an identity check is sometimes useful. A review of the modern history of public psychiatry leads to the identification of several axes that, taken together as a profile, help to characterize and explain the modern and contemporary periods. Variation on each axis tends to be cyclical. The axes include:

(1) narrow (pre-community mental health and system development) versus broad definitions of the target population (community mental health and mainstreaming);

(2) segregation of mental health services and systems theory (state hospitals and community services development) versus integration into medical and social services and benefits (community mental health and mainstreaming);

(3) delineation of boundaries (pre-community mental health and community services development) versus blurring of public/private domains (mainstreaming);

(4) clinical structures (community mental health) versus corporate, cost and organizational structures (mainstreaming);

(5) paternal attitudes (asylums) versus patient rights and autonomy (community mental health and later periods);

(6) state versus federal responsibility and funding;

(7) treatment tasks (community mental health) versus responsibility for social control (community services development and later);

(8) science (since community mental health) versus ideology (pre-community mental health and psychoanalysis) and, to complete a profile,

(9) optimism (community mental health) versus pessimism (pre-community mental health).

Use of these axes, analogous to use of the Minnesota Multiphasic Personality Inventory (MMPI) for a single person, provides an interesting, synthetic profile of public psychiatry at the current time.

At present, the field of public psychiatry finds itself in:

(1) a time of broad definition of target population;
(2) a fragmented system;
(3) a period of invigorated mainstreaming;
(4) a blurring of public and private boundaries;
(5) a culture of business strategies for the purpose of cost control (versus professional and clinical principles);
(6) a rise in autonomy for individuals with illness as the prevailing philosophy;
(7) a partnership of state and federal authority;
(8) a balance of professional and social control roles for some categorical populations while swinging back to professional treatment roles for physicians and, in the circumstances of much ferment about the future, with
(9) a mixture of discouragement—related to the slow progress of clinical practice and budget constraints—and optimism—rooted in the potential of health care reform to expand nondiscriminatory mental health insurance, transformation, and scientific research to lead psychiatry out of a challenging time.

Health care reform and other variables shaping the future of public psychiatry will shift the field of practice on most of these axes.

FACTORS IN THE EQUATION OF CHANGE FOR PUBLIC PSYCHIATRY

It is possible to identify multiple factors that already are shaping the future or have the potential to shape public psychiatry over the next several years. Table 8-1 lists them in no particular order.

All the factors identified in the table have been introduced previously in chapters 6 and 7. It is necessary to keep an eye on all of them. However, by far, health care reform passed in 2010 dominates the scene and incorporates many of the other variables.

HEALTH CARE REFORM UNDER THE PPAC ACT

Health care reform was the leading political and legislative agenda of the Obama Administration. It takes aim at the entire health care system and holds far-reaching significance for public psychiatry in particular. The scale of the PPAC Act of 2010 dwarfs the presidential commissions on

Table 8-1 Variables Shaping Change in Public Psychiatry

- Transformation
  - Integration of mental health into primary care
  - Consumer and family driven mental health care (person-centered care)
  - Elimination of disparities in health care outcomes
  - Routine early screening and referral to mental health services
  - Excellent mental health care via evidence-based practices
  - Personal health information systems and electronic medical records
  - Acute care crisis
- Recovery
  - Empowerment
  - Person-centered planning of care
  - Peer services
- Translation of discoveries, evidence-based practice
- Health care reform (the PPAC Act)
  - Parity of insurance
  - Expanded insurance coverage
  - Changes in Medicaid
  - Cost control and accountability
  - Changes in reimbursement
  - Quality (regulatory review)
  - Deinstitutionalization of nursing homes
- Community-based forensic clinical services
  - Deinstitutionalization
  - Transitional clinical services
- General, medical issues
  - Patient safety
  - Quality of care
  - Patient-centered, medical homes
- Social problems
  - Homelessness
- Politics and economics
  - Economic recession
  - National and state elections
  - National and state fiscal crises

mental health during the past half century. The timeline for implementation of PPAC is nine years. Given concerns about cost and impact on the federal deficit, Congress will probably revisit and modify the legislation over the next several years. Insurers and managed care companies will have a say through litigation that challenges some of its provisions. Even as the PPAC Act is subject to revision and challenge, it is still useful to begin to understand it and its implications for public psychiatry.

Three themes dominated the public debate of health care reform over the year prior to enactment. They were (a) expansion of access to healthcare, (b) control of health care costs and federal spending, and (c) improvement in the quality of health care. All three have implications for the future of public psychiatry and medicine in general.

The PPAC Act expands access to behavioral health care by covering 32 million uninsured people (some estimates are 30 million). The basic, health benefit package includes nondiscriminatory benefits for mental and substance-use disorders. This feature reinforces previously enacted parity legislation (in 2008) that established nondiscriminatory behavioral health insurance coverage in Medicare and commercial insurance. The combination of expanded access to uninsured people and behavioral benefits at parity creates a powerful dynamic for expanding demand for services. As a result, demand for behavioral health services probably burgeons in both the private and public domains of psychiatry. In policy briefs sent out during 2009 and 2010, the National Council of Community Behavioral Health roughly estimated a 50% increase in the number of people expecting to be served in the current publicly funded, private nonprofit sector.

The expansion of access is not created by categorical funding of new, special programs, but rather by building on existing commercial insurance and entitlement programs. Reimbursement from these payers establishes new revenue streams to providers of service, who can then expand services to meet the new demand. Of central importance to public psychiatry, Medicaid plays a key role in expansion of access to care, though not until 2014 (see below).

The need to control health care costs, as well as to protect the viability of expanded access, requires that the new access go hand-in-hand with accountability by providers. Utilization management of care intensifies for all providers of service, including those in the public sector. Thorough documentation of services and efficient billing for services become essential for agencies to maintain revenue streams. In addition, incentives to develop prevention, to coordinate care, and to reduce duplication of services are part of cost control. Productivity grows as a concern in order to maintain balanced provider budgets. Further, instead of fee-for-service, the new landscape includes bundled, capitated, and performance-based reimbursement mechanisms, in order to change practice patterns, share risk, improve quality, and control costs. In short, the administrative requirement related to these measures poses strong challenges for service agencies in public psychiatry.

Quality is a counterpoint to cost control. It is part of the equation for computing the value of services. To work with the equation, payers require health care providers to measure, monitor, and report the outcomes of their services. Incentives to implement evidence-based, effective interventions also intensify. Also, in response to the quality agenda, providers need to efficiently translate new discoveries into practice. Further, the Joint Commission on Accreditation of Healthcare Organizations and other accreditation agencies contribute to in the pursuit of quality of care. Through random and unannounced site visits, regulatory bodies keep institutions on their toes. A focus on quality aims at improvement of the value of care. Continuous quality improvement is already part of administrative and clinical operations in public psychiatry. It can only grow and may be a challenge for some.

In summary, health care reform is a combination of increased access, augmented accountability and an intensified quality of care. Services must develop a consumer orientation in order to build revenue streams and expand. In order to participate and comply with the new system, investment in computerized systems is necessary. Budgets that have been predicated largely on grants from state mental health authorities become revenue-based and require a different kind of fiscal management. In a variety of ways, the three-part package of health care reform, while offering opportunities to behavioral health agencies in public psychiatry, poses enormous leadership and administrative challenges for them as well.

MEDICAID UNDER THE PPAC ACT

Under the PPAC Act, Medicaid plays an essential role in the expansion of access to health care for low income people. It is estimated that Medicaid will cover 16 million new people by 2019, about half of the population of uninsured at present (Kaiser Family Foundation, 2010b). For the most part, the new enrollees are dependent children and adults, without children, under the age of 65. Many of the new services are channeled through federally qualified community health centers (CHCs). CHCs have played a long, successful role in providing access to health care for low income people. They receive expanded support under the PPAC Act. In response to demand for services, CHCs are likely to expand their role in mental health services, not only through demonstration projects of integrated primary care, but also through revenue based expansion of behavioral capacity predicated on their cost-based reimbursement under Medicaid.

The benefit package for the new enrollees in Medicaid is a benchmark package that does not include special supportive and enabling services for high-need populations. Special services for people with serious mental illness, who are typically served by public psychiatry, include long-term care, psychosocial rehabilitation, and case management. Medicaid continues to support these special services for presently enrolled elderly and disabled people. Presumably, to the extent that new enrollees meet criteria of eligibility for the special services, they will be able to access these services, too. Also, under PPAC, chronic disease management programs include severe and persistent mental disorders among the chronic diseases that receive attention. As these programs develop, yet another kind of service may become available to this high-need population.

The dually eligible population is a Medicaid group that receives special attention under PPAC. Low income, elderly and disabled people who are on Medicare and also receive Medicaid as an adjunct benefit to help pay for Medicare premiums and services not covered by Medicare, are known as "dual eligibles." The combined benefits continue for this population. The dual population comprised 18% of Medicaid enrollees and accounted for 46% of Medicaid expenditures in 2005. The PPAC Act creates an office to coordinate care for dual eligibles. It also contains provisions to encourage states to develop "community first" options, in part through chronic disease management programs. Reciprocally, PPAC invests in special needs programs (SNPs) for chronically ill people under Medicare, which by 2012 have to contract with Medicaid. People with severe and persistent mental illness also are eligible for these programs. Over time, these initiatives are designed to control Medicaid nursing home costs. Indeed, insofar as nursing homes serve as sites for most institutional chronic care of people with serious mental illness, this program under Medicaid through Money Follows the Person mechanisms, has the potential to fundamentally redesign this part of the public mental health system. It is a new wave of deinstitutionalization for people with serious mental illness.

It is important to point out that the PPAC Act contains multiple other Medicaid initiatives. These are:

(1) medical home pilot studies;
(2) development of peer services;
(3) emergency care pilots regarding institutions for mental disorders (IMDs);
(4) pilots of pediatric accountable care organization, and
(5) bundled reimbursement demonstration projects (National Council for Community Behavioral Health, 2010b).

Pilot studies of medical homes figures in the evolving integration of mental health into primary care. Funding of peer services supports an important development that comes out of the transformation agenda. The emergency care pilots presumably address emergency room gridlock and may expand access to acute care, thereby relieving the existing acute care crisis. The discussion below picks up these initiatives.

The changes in Medicaid continue to shift the locus of policy and program action from state departments of mental health to state Medicaid agencies. Medicaid has grown in importance for financing mental health services over the past two decades. It helped shape a community services system for people with serious mental illness after the community mental health movement. During periods of fiscal stringency related to multiple economic recessions since 1982, many states pursued services backed by matching Medicaid reimbursement. The federal matching assistance percentage (FMAP) helped states to control general fund expenditures while developing services. In 2006, Medicaid costs, including both general fund and FMAP matching reimbursement, were the largest line item in state budgets by a slight margin of 21.5% versus 21.4% for K-12 education (Georgetown University Health Policy Institute, 2008). Under PPAC, some place Medicaid as high as 335% by 2035 (Open Minds, 2010). Thus, when expansion of access under health care reform is complete, Medicaid would have an even more preeminent role in funding public psychiatric services.

NOT ONLY POLITICS BUT ALSO ECONOMICS

The fiscal crises of states subsequent to the national financial crash and recession of 2008 considerably affects the transition to the new financing of behavioral health care under the PPHCA Act. Most states face cumulative budget deficits of multibillions of dollars over the three years since 2008. Connecticut, for example, faced an $8 billion shortfall over the budget biennium starting July 1, 2009. Already states are beginning to trim public mental health services (Rosenberg, 2009). The timetable for implementation of the PPAC Act is not synchronized with this fiscal crisis in the states. In some cases, states may cut services before alternative funding is in place. In other cases, privatization is a strategy. States such as New Jersey, Georgia, California, and Connecticut, to mention a few, are already considering privatization of human services such as group homes, state owned hospitals, and other special services.

In most statehouses, as a result of growth in Medicaid as a budgetary line item, Medicaid is a target for the purposes of budget control and deficit reduction. This was the case from 2001 to 2004 because of state budget deficits. It is the case again, and can only intensify as federal stimulus money runs out in 2011. During the Bush administration, as a prelude to a Medicaid Reform Commission, Congress passed the Deficit Reduction Act (DRA) of 2006, which introduced new flexibility for states to change the traditional nature of Medicaid. The tools given to states to pursue reform included "limited benefit" and "fixed contribution" plans. It is uncertain how the combination of the fiscal pressure and state flexibility to define mandated and optional benefits is going to play out.

Medicaid optional benefits may become a target (Rosenberg, 2009). These benefits have traditionally supported services for people with serious mental illness. The state of Michigan has already targeted optional benefits. States may retrench to basic benchmark acute care benefit packages in order to compensate for the costs of increased access to the entitlement. As a result, community support programs, assertive community treatment, and case management now reimbursed as optional benefits could suffer. If retrenchment on optional benefits reimbursed by Medicaid proves true, the question of who supports rehabilitation, long-term care, and support services in the community turns urgent. The logical place to turn would be state mental health authorities that have played a traditional role for over a century in caring for individuals with serious mental illness.

Experience from the economic recession that began in 2008, which was the last of five economic downturns since 1972, emphasizes the importance of economic and fiscal issues as underlying themes in the evolution of public psychiatry. Major recessions were associated with the transition from community mental health to community services development, from community services development to mainstreaming, and from mainstreaming to transformation. Though it is hard to fully anticipate the implications for public psychiatry of the current recession, which is the worst since 1932, it most likely serves as a significant brake on the forces of expansion under health care reform. Also, the current economic challenges requires an intensification of accountability and cost control as part of health care reform.

STATE DEPARTMENTS OF MENTAL HEALTH AND THE PPAC ACT

The policy directions under PPAC hold important implications for state mental health authorities and community mental health centers in the public arena. Reciprocally, as state Medicaid agencies have considerably expanded roles secondary to Medicaid expansion, state departments of mental health have reduced, and residual, roles.

Indeed, one scenario for state mental health authorities is involution and disappearance over time as implementation of the PPAC progresses. The logic of this scenario depends largely on how, after PPAC, the residual uninsured population of about 15 million people is served. The disappearance of state mental health authorities, which have traditionally served the uninsured in each state, would be contingent on the convergence of several developments. If CHCs step up to an enhanced role in mental health under PPAC, thereby expanding access under Medicaid, it would support this direction. If private nonprofit community mental health centers achieve federally qualified status through the Mental Health and Addictions Safety Net Equity Act (HR5636), which was introduced into Congress in 2110 by Representatives Matsue (D-Cal) and Engle (D-NY), then it also would support this direction. Federal qualification would potentially enhance their reimbursement rates but also require that they serve the residual uninsured population. Finally, as states face up to the costs of Medicaid expansion, if they shift their traditional safety net responsibility for uninsured, mentally ill people through their state mental health authorities to local community-based health and mental health agencies, it will push in this direction. As a corollary, in order to take advantage of the FMAP, states would offer whatever mental health services they provide through Medicaid. The net result of all these would be the transfer of a traditional state responsibility to community-based, private nonprofit agencies, which are given federal incentives. This perfect storm of developments could lead to obsolescence of the state mental health authorities in their present incarnation.

> The net result of all these would be the transfer of a traditional state responsibility to community-based, private nonprofit agencies.

On the other hand, the following scenario seems more likely. State departments of mental health probably retain several residual and special roles. These include partial responsibility for mental health services for the 15 million people in the United States, who remain uninsured after implementation of PPAC. In addition, these departments may administer special long-term care and rehabilitative services for the new enrollees in Medicaid under the PPAC Act—either pending eligibility determinations for long-term care benefits under Medicaid, or for Medicare enrollees who are not eligible for Medicaid, i.e., non-dually eligible people. Management of residential resources for people with serious mental illness probably would continue, especially as these resources become the main platform for community-based care still managed by state mental health authorities. Finally, special forensic clinical services remain and constitute one of the main responsibilities of state mental health agencies (see below). Nevertheless, the net result of these speculations is a considerable reconfiguration of the profile of clinical programs in the domain of public psychiatry under the direction of state mental health authorities.

Neither the expansion of insurance coverage nor mainstreaming of mental health benefits under Medicaid attends to maintenance of the system of services presently under state mental health authorities. For three decades, state owned and operated services and state networks of private nonprofit local mental health authorities, which receive grants from the state, have made up the public system. In the new scheme, state plans for Medicaid, including state choices of options such as home health care, which is administered under state Medicaid agencies, replace the system functions of the departments of mental health. As a consequence, state departments of mental health need to work out consulting and advisory relationships with the Medicaid agencies in their states, which typically have neither extensive nor deeply experienced behavioral health expertise. For example, the emphasis of health care reform on improved access through health insurance for acute care might strengthen a narrowly defined model of medical and psychiatric care that gives short shrift to long-term care for chronic diseases. Psychiatric disorders, at least in the public sector, are severe and persistent. Chronic, recurrent, disabling psychiatric disorders are an essential focus for effective public psychiatric practice. Given these considerations, state mental health authorities may need to move in to fill gaps in chronic care with services they traditionally have provided.

COMMUNITY MENTAL HEALTH CENTERS AND HEALTH REFORM

The PPAC Act changes the definition of community mental health centers to require that their payer mix includes at least 40% of the population that is ineligible for Medicare. Also, it provides $50 million for co-location of primary and specialty care in community-based behavioral health, administered by the SAMHSA. Furthermore, there may be an opportunity for community mental health centers to qualify as patient- (person-) centered health homes for people with serious mental illness insofar as they are the principal caregivers for this population.

The enormous expansion in access to behavioral insurance benefits under PPAC has the potential to substantially increase demand for behavioral services. The new definition of community mental health centers assumes they play a role in providing incremental access. The expansion of services in response to demand would create new revenue streams for private nonprofit community mental health centers. Inasmuch as new revenue streams are the formula for expansion, state owned and operated community mental health centers probably will play a minor, if not diminishing, role in the future. Even the future role of independent private nonprofit community mental health centers is not clear. It seems likely that CHCs might dominate new developments. This is true because they play a critical role in integrated primary care for people with serious mental illness and have advantageous, cost-based reimbursement under Medicaid. Also, CHCs are earmarked for expanded funding under the PPCA Act, given their traditional role and track record in providing access to low income people. Community mental health centers, unless they achieve federally qualified status, may find it attractive, if not essential, to affiliate or merge with CHCs.

INTEGRATION OF PRIMARY AND BEHAVIORAL HEALTH CARE

Health care reform incorporates and carries forward a number of goals from the transformation agenda. These include integrated primary care, recovery, and measures to address the acute care crisis.

The challenge of improving life expectancy among people with serious mental illness is the leading public health task for psychiatry today. In 2006, the National Association of State Mental Health Program Directors (NASMHPD) documented a 25-year shortened life expectancy for people with serious mental illness (NASMHPD, 2006). As a result, the national Center for Disease Control (CDC) began to monitor mortality for this high-risk group. The solution to the problem requires community mental health centers to integrate with primary care. In a sense, it is the reciprocal of the dictum that there is no health with mental health.

Two main platforms are possible for offering primary care to people with serious mental illness. One is the primary care clinic. CHCs, because of their cost-based reimbursement, discounted pharmacy procurement, and low overhead as a result of construction grants and liability protection, are the leading candidates for addressing the problem from this direction.

The other platform for integration is community mental health centers, which are the principal caregivers for many people with serious mental illness. If Senate Bill 2182 is enacted, community mental health centers may be eligible to become person-centered medical homes for people with SMI. The PPHA Act provides for pilot studies of community mental health centers as medical homes. Also, private nonprofit community mental health centers (but not state owned and operated ones) may have the opportunity to apply to the Health Resources and Services Administration (HRSA) to become federally qualified health center (CHC) "look-alikes," thereby improving their reimbursement for both medical and mental health care. A vehicle for achieving this integration at the level of clinical care is person-centered health care, an evidence-based consumer empowerment practice. It fosters integration on the level of the individual patient and brings clinicians of behavioral health and primary care together in a single plan of care.

Though SAMHSA launched a "10 by 10" public awareness program (improvement by 10 years of shortened life expectancy by 2010), success in pursuit of this goal will take years. Not just clinical care but also prevention and wellness programs make an essential contribution to success in meeting this goal. Recognizing this challenge, in spring 2009 SAMHSA issued a request for proposals for seven demonstration projects. The appropriation bills of FY210 and the PPAC Act expanded the funding of these demonstrations, which double the number of sites with demonstration projects. Because it is a conspicuous public health problem that the Centers for Disease Control now monitors, this task endures as a powerful force for change in the field of public psychiatry.

RECOVERY AND PERSON-CENTERED CARE

Recovery in psychiatry is part of a larger movement in medicine for people with cancer and other chronic diseases to improve care by making them active participants in treatment and "owners" of their care. It remains a powerful organizing concept for transforming the service system. In 2008, the Centers for Medicare and Medicaid (CMS) awarded a contract to investigators at the CMHC to implement person-centered care planning throughout Connecticut. This evidence-based practice incorporates recovery concepts into practice, giving the recipient of care an active role in care planning. Person-centered care introduces into the process of care goals related to living and working in the community. This clinical vehicle provides a concrete strategy for implementing recovery in public psychiatry. Once strategies and procedures are worked out under this contract, the practice can be extended across the United States.

The ramifications of recovery on the process of care are manifold. Under the broad rubric of recovery, burden of disease enters into the equation of care. With an eye on recovery, it is no longer enough to treat symptoms; it is also essential to prevent and reduce disability. More effective use of treatment and rehabilitative modalities, and their integration, serve this goal. Recovery is not possible if mentally ill people do not attend to their physical health or if they are ill with chronic medical problems. For this reason, recovery calls for an integration of behavioral health and primary care. Also, "peers" who are themselves in recovery from mental illness have a role to play in supporting, coaching and guiding others like themselves in the course of illness and treatment in the mental health system. These roles cement their active participation in and responsibility for their own care. Multiple powerful implications such as these argue for the durability of recovery as a variable for changing public psychiatry. Furthermore, the PPAC Act gives impetus to peer services by supporting their development.

THE ACUTE CARE CRISIS

The acute care crisis is manifest in the gridlock that exists in general hospital emergency rooms and on hospital inpatient units. The growing acute care crisis was the topic of a 2003 subcommittee report of the NFC. It was also the topic of an influential American Hospital Association (AHA) report that appeared in 2007. In response to the mounting difficulties of general hospitals in Connecticut, a governor's commission made recommendations the same year. While the reasons for the problem are multiple and complex, a fundamental issue is the underpayment by Medicaid and state contracts for general hospital-level services. Further, in the face of budget crises over the years, most state governments have cut back on hospital beds as they stretch their resources to support community-based care as a priority. General hospitals have become de facto parts of the public service system. They are in an untenable fiscal position, and many have eliminated their psychiatric beds.

The AHA report provides a framework for addressing this problem. One centerpiece idea is to bring together the parties involved in the crisis—including general hospitals, community mental health centers, city and state government authorities, and recipients of care—to work out a local system solution. The analysis of the problem and the solution will vary from community to community. In analysis of data from a series of meetings in New Haven, Connecticut, a work group concluded that the problem is one of (a) inadequate step-down resources for people leaving acute care, (b) inadequate alternatives to hospitalization, and (c) inadequate triage of people in crisis away from the emergency rooms of the two general hospitals. As a general proposition the general hospitals accepted responsibility for acute care in the emergency room and hospital but wanted more efficient community-based services from the public mental health and substance abuse systems. Also, they wanted closer collaboration between the private and public sectors in order to address the crisis. The consequences of this process in New Haven means tighter integration of acute care in hospitals with a spectrum of community-based services as alternatives to hospitalization, facilitation of step-down from the hospital, and prevention of relapse. This results in a resetting of priorities in the public mental health system, which has functioned independently for the most part, following principles inherent to traditional community mental health care. Central among the new goals is to make more efficient and effective use of expensive hospital resources by orienting to patients in emergency rooms and coming out of hospital units.

The evolution of public psychiatry in response to the acute care crisis takes place on a local level and varies from community to community depending on local circumstances. While much of the discussion above is parochial to New Haven, similar system development will occur across the country, as no region is immune to the crisis. Resolution of the acute care crisis becomes a major part of mainstreaming mental health services into close alignment with medical care and services. Both the solution to the acute care crisis and the integration of behavioral and primary care services, discussed above, converge in a tighter relationship between public psychiatry and medical services.

The expansion of mental health insurance benefits, which takes place over several years, and the implementation of parity, which goes forward in 2010, may go a long way to resolving the existing acute care crisis (depending on reimbursement levels) by providing income to hospitals for care that is now undercompensated or uncompensated. Also, Medicaid under PPAC supports pilot studies for IMDs to reorient themselves to (and demonstrate a role in) acute care. The redirected resources can help alleviate the shortage of beds.

> The expansion of mental health insurance benefits and the implementation of parity may resolve the existing acute care crisis.

EARLY INTERVENTION IN FIRST-EPISODE PSYCHOSIS

One of the main goals of the NFC report of 2003 was to refocus attention on the early stages of illness for the sake of preventing chronic symptoms and disability. The PPAC Act is silent on this issue. In part, the NFC recommendation aimed to reduce the large expenses associated with intractable illness late in the course of disease. A leading example of early intervention is the demonstration grant from the National Institute of Mental Health (NIMH) to implement and evaluate, through a national consortium, early intervention for people with first episodes of psychosis. The importance of this demonstration is evident in the $80 million dollar budget. This massive demonstration, known as Recovery After Initial Schizophrenic Episodes (RAISE), has the power to transform the treatment of schizophrenic illness.

The concept of early intervention harkens back to central ideas of the community mental health movement. It is intuitively convincing in a theoretical framework derived from public health. However, early intervention in initial episodes of psychosis is still unproven. In order to achieve the potential of the idea, much needs to be done. Obviously, data from the demonstration project must be collected and analyzed to document the effectiveness of the approach in reducing burden of disease and costs of care. Even so, more effort is needed in the form of advocacy for health insurance benefits to cover the elements of care in an early intervention program. With success in obtaining reimbursement, there would be incentive for community mental health centers and mental health clinics in CHCs to implement the services. Having accomplished these steps, there is the potential of early intervention to reduce disability and burden of disease for people with schizophrenic illness and their families.

COMMUNITY-BASED FORENSIC SERVICES

Federal and state demonstration grants for services to people who are exiting prisons already have begun to configure the service profile of public psychiatry as well as expand the population to be served. States, which are under pressure to reduce budget deficits, may revise their policies on incarceration of offenders for drug use and minor offenses, eventually leading to a flood of releases (Steinhauer, 2009). Also, the federal Second Chance Act of 2008 is likely to accelerate the exodus from prisons. As a result, this special population of people in need of service may grow exponentially. The question is whether the development of special, categorical services can keep up with the flow of people in need. Community mental health and addiction services, despite categorical funding, already are filling the demand for services from people exiting prison or have been diverted by courts. The demand for service requires community mental health centers and clinics to reorient toward the need, sometimes through specific newly funded categorical programs, and sometimes from existing resources. Over time, in concert with the migration of acute clinical services to CHCs and private nonprofit agencies under PPAC, it is possible that community forensic services will grow to become the largest program of services for state departments of mental health.

SERVICES FOR PEOPLE WITH SERIOUS MENTAL ILLNESS IN THE FUTURE

During the almost five-decade era of modern of public psychiatry at the CMHC, various movements and legislative initiatives have developed a wide array of services and benefits in the community as an alternative to long-term hospitalization (see Table 8-2). No single period got it all right. Rather, it is the accumulation of services accrued in different phases of modern development that accounts for the current picture. More recent services, such as peer services and integrated primary care, need consolidation over more time. A transition is presently in play that leads from procrustean programs of service, offered practically to everyone, to person-centered care, where elements of service are mobilized into individualized plans of care. Consumer empowerment, control, and choice support this change. Also, the picture portrayed in the table is not complete. Home-based services for dually eligible people under PPAC hold promise as a whole new range of services that can help deinstitutionalize chronically ill people now in nursing homes. This iteration of the table, which has been used in previous chapters to portray a growing spectrum of services, includes a column indicating the status of the service in the future.

There is a need to sustain all the services to provide the range of options required by individuals at different points in the trajectory of serious and persistent mental illness. At the same time, public psychiatry faces the recurrent fundamental problem of insufficient resources. Few of the services are totally secure going forward. Some are in greater jeopardy of budget cuts, or even elimination, if effort is not made to defend them. In Table 8-2, the services that seem most in jeopardy, by virtue of budget cutbacks, redefinitions of benefit packages, or reduced roles for state mental health authorities, are identified in the right-hand column. The number of services identified as at risk suggests there is a major agenda ahead to maintain an array of services through the current economic recession and health care reform. The responsibility to monitor and advocate for services for people with severe and persistent mental illness is part of an ongoing obligation to establish a priority for the "least well off" in the circumstances of mainstreaming and health care reform (Goldman, 1999).

Given the limited resources related to concerns about the cost of health care reform and the need of entitlements to restrain expenditures, it appears necessary to set service priorities for the public system in order that the most needy and vulnerable are not lost and left behind. Can

Table 8-2 Service Type or Benefit by Period in Modern Public Psychiatry: The Future of Services for People With Serious Mental Illness

Service Type or Benefit	Post–WW II	CMH	CSS	Main	Trans	Future
Asylum, chronic hospitalization	X					needed
Acute inpatient hospitalization		X	X	X	X	crisis
Nursing home, long-term care		X	X	X	X	changing under PPAC
Partial hospitalization, intensive outpatient			X	X	X	more needed
Routine outpatient, ambulatory care		X	X	X	X	
Emergency room	X	X	X	X	X	crisis
Urgent care		X	X	X	X	
Crisis intervention		X	X	X	X	more needed
Neighborhood clinics		X				
Prevention, early intervention		X			X	needed
Assertive community treatment			X	X	X	changing
Co-occurring services					X	unclear
Vocational rehabilitation			X	X	X	
Psychosocial rehabilitation	X		X	X	X	
Case management, community support programs			X	X	X	changing
Residential services			X	X	X	
System development, local mental health authorities			X	X	X	waning
Outreach to homeless				X	X	
Medicaid Medicare		X	X	X	X	changing under PPAC
Recovery, quality of life goals					X	more needed

Table 8-2 (Continued)						
Service Type or Benefit	**Post–WW II**	**CMH**	**CSS**	**Main**	**Trans**	**Future**
Peer services					X	more needed
Integrated primary medical care					X	integration under way
Supplemental Security Income Social Security Disability Insurance		X	X	X	X	

Abbreviations: CMH, Community Mental Health; CSS, Community Services and Systems; Main, Mainstreaming; Post–WW II, Post–World War II; Trans, Transformation.

some services be relegated to the new revenue-based service paradigm? Can some be consolidated? For instance, do systems need to sustain separate programs of assertive community treatment and community support or might they combine the two and develop procedures to identify and provide more intensive care for those who are in crisis? Over the next few years, the public system will grapple with such issues.

THE DEFINITION AND PRACTICE OF PUBLIC PSYCHIATRY IN THE FUTURE

The introduction in chapter 1 offered a working definition of public psychiatry for the purpose of orientation to the narrative. Over the course of this historical account, that definition seems to stand the test of time, especially its emphasis on payers. Still, though the definition is not in need of fundamental revision, the contemporary scene suggests changes in emphasis for considering future directions in public psychiatry. On the broadest level—the change in character of the population served by public psychiatry—vigilance is needed to preserve balanced use of resources and programs within institutions for people with serious mental illness. Also, given the prominence of social problems in American society, public psychiatrists require knowledge of forensic practice and of roles that are a function of social control, versus clinical roles, in psychiatric practice. These include reporting to criminal justice authorities or exercising civil commitment procedures, and Tarasoff responsibilities when reaching out to homeless or managing behavior as part of services to forensic populations. The acute care crisis suggests the possibility of further subspecialization in roles for the private and public sectors. Thus, general hospitals will focus on acute care. Public facilities will focus on triage, crisis care, alternatives to hospitalization such as respite care, and step-down levels of care, including a full spectrum of residential placements. Public practice in the future requires integration with primary care and clinical consultation roles on services co-located in primary care sites. In addition, public psychiatrists need to know basic health promotion and be able to monitor high-risk conditions such as obesity, metabolic syndrome, and chronic conditions such as diabetes and hypertension in mental health sites. Under the PPAC Act, the location of services undergoes a major shift. In the future, private nonprofit agencies will expand, continuing a process already under way in many states; state owned and operated services retrench; and CHCs have the potential to expand enormously. It is conceivable, given the need to co-locate services to integrate mental health and primary care that the main locus of public psychiatry will migrate to CHCs.

Though the question of privatizing services has receded in intensity since the time of privatization and managed care in the previous decade, it still might be a reasonable strategy for many policy makers and legislators looking in on public psychiatry from the outside. In a broader perspective, it is true that much of public psychiatry has already migrated over the past 30 years to a private nonprofit, both hospital and ambulatory, sphere. States now routinely contract with general hospitals for most acute hospital care. On the other hand, health care reform, mainstreaming, and attenuation of a system of care for people with serious mental illness, as well as expansion of other target populations of public psychiatry, make it all the more necessary to have state mental health authorities and psychiatric professionals concerned about patients and services in the public sector. In the absence of a system, much will depend on clinical process. On a system level, Drs. David Frank and Sherry Glied argue the need for coordination of federal and state agencies for the purpose of integrating public mental health policy (Frank and Glied, 2006).

A focus on serving people with serious mental illness has a cyclical pattern in the modern era, reaching a high point in the years of community services and system development after the community mental health movement. Perhaps for no other reason, American society needs presidential commissions every 20 years or so to renew its commitment. In any event, historical precedent and objective need on a clinical level argue for individuals with serious and persistent illness as a cornerstone group in the target population of public psychiatry. In the circumstances where the population served by public psychiatry has expanded considerably over the periods of mainstreaming and transformation, it may no longer be possible to define clearly a target population. Usually this exercise is done in the circumstances of budget deficits and for the purpose of setting priorities. More helpful than a diffuse definition of target population would be a listing of populations served by the public sector and then setting priorities for the general fund dollars. It is arguable that individuals with serious mental illness ought to be at the top of this list of priorities. Furthermore, given the proliferation of categorically funded programs and new revenue streams for acute care under PPAC, hard pressed general fund dollars might be reserved for programs such as psychosocial rehabilitation and residential programs that serve the needs of people with serious and persistent mental illness.

EDUCATION IN PUBLIC PSYCHIATRY IN THE FUTURE

Chapter 1, with a definition of public psychiatry under discussion, indicated this book would return to the question of education. Here, given consideration of services and practice in public psychiatry over the modern era, the stage is set to contend that public psychiatry is a specialized type of psychiatric practice. Under health care reform and other factors shaping practice in public psychiatry, including mainstreaming and diminution of mental health system functions, it is all the more important to have dedicated, specialized professionals in public psychiatry.

A cogent argument can be made for advanced, subspecialty board certified training in public psychiatry. In recent years, two groups have made the case for such training (Brown et al., 1993; Yedida et al., 2006). One, representing the American Association of Community Psychiatrists, defined the clinical, consultative, administrative and academic components, including the knowledge, skills, competencies, and structure for this special education (Brown et al., 1993). The other, representing a distinguished public psychiatry education program at Columbia University, recently described the elements of public psychiatry training essential to education in the field (Ranz et al., 2008). There are notable, long-standing education programs in public psychiatry. They include those in the departments of psychiatry at Columbia University, University of Massachusetts, University of Colorado, the University of Oregon, the University of Maryland, and Yale University.

Psychiatric residents are not well prepared for public psychiatry in their general psychiatric education. At the same time, there are a growing number of psychiatrists who work at least part time in the public arena (Ranz et al., 2006). A recent study surveyed psychiatry residency programs and discovered that many—despite recognizing the need and significance—fail to meet objectives of importance in public psychiatry education, particularly in regard to cross-institutional integration of services (Yedida et al., 2006). Development of special education programs would fill an existing need and be a bridge to the future.

In the past 25 years or so, psychiatry has witnessed the development of several subspecialties. These include addictions, forensic psychiatry, consultation psychiatry, emergency psychiatry, and geriatric psychiatry. All of these have special educational requirements. It is clear that public psychiatrists also require specialized education in order to practice competently and effectively. For example, public psychiatrists must understand psychiatric disability and know how to complete functional assessments. They must also be knowledgeable about psychosocial and vocational rehabilitation in order to integrate these interventions into comprehensive plans of care. They should appreciate the principle of recovery, know best practices such as person-centered care, and should be at ease in their interactions with recipients of care so as to respond sympathetically and effectively to their needs and aspirations. Public psychiatrists must know how to collaborate with other community-based professionals, who provide residential and money management services that support people outside the hospital. They must be competent, if not qualified, in the evaluation and treatment of addiction disorders. They should have a working understanding of legal problems commonly encountered by people seeking services in the public sector. Psychiatrists working in the public arena must be effective members of interdisciplinary teams, often as clinical team leaders, and confident about medical roles in both clinical and community settings, while also remaining aware of the roles of other professional groups. They must understand how nontraditional mechanisms of care are employed beyond the walls of the clinic for the purpose of reaching out and serving people who are homeless or unable to attend appointments on a regular basis. Finally, psychiatrists in public settings optimally achieve an understanding of organizations, systems, system dynamics, management, leadership, and a population perspective on psychiatric disorders and the application of clinical resources.

Professionals base their practice on scientific and clinical bodies of knowledge, as well as theories derived from them, which through testing lead to revised knowledge. Public psychiatrists as professionals have over time based their practice on evolving theories and knowledge bases. Central to the beginning of the modern era of public and community psychiatry was a public health model, offering the advantage of roots in the sciences of epidemiology and services research. Systems theory and sociopolitical theories were also important building blocks at the beginning. Preclinical and clinical science, including attention to biological, psychological, and social variables, were a cornerstone of practice. All of these contributed to, and enhanced, a broad medical model for conceptualizing practice. Biopsychosocial systems theory emerged as a prominent model in the second decade of the modern era before the field of psychiatry veered toward a narrow, biological paradigm over the past 25 years. There is a dialogue among community psychiatrists, continuing to the present, regarding medical science and knowledge versus humanistic philosophy, including personal and political liberation goals (Cohen et al., 2003). As a function of the transformation agenda, there is a return to some of the roots of the modern public psychiatry movement, emphasizing again a public health model, while continuing to affirm a commitment to humanistic values (American Association of Community Psychiatrists, 2007).

Psychiatrists interested in public psychiatry identify with one or more of a few national associations for professional development. These include the American Association of Community Psychiatrists (AACP), the American Association of Social Psychiatry, the American Orthopsychiatry Association, and the Radical Caucus of members of the American Psychiatric Association. An important professional journal for the public psychiatrist is the *Community Mental Health Journal*, which the AACP publishes. In addition, public psychiatrists regularly contribute to and read *Psychiatric Services* and, to a lesser extent, the *Journal of Orthopsychiatry*, not to mention general psychiatric journals.

There is no doubt that public psychiatry makes important contributions to academic departments of psychiatry. Another volume has considered the contributions to public psychiatry of academic programs at the CMHC (Jacobs and Griffith, 2007). The establishment of advanced qualifications in public psychiatry would only enhance these contributions. Also, advanced qualifications would support and consolidate a cadre of professionals who are needed to take the field of public psychiatry forward in a time of great change.

THE FUTURE OF SERVICES AND ACADEMIC MISSIONS AT THE CMHC

Leading to a conclusion, this section turns from general consideration of future directions for public psychiatry to the particular case of the

CMHC. Consideration of the variables shaping future directions in public psychiatry portend important shifts in character for the CMHC but no radical change in the fundamental mission of the institution. Of note as background, Connecticut has not aggressively "medicaided" its mental health services, and in comparison to many states still expends substantial state dollars on state owned and operated services. For example, the state still operates a small (and reduced) number of acute care beds and funds many long-term care services out of its general fund. Also, the state owns, operates, and supports five community mental health centers. The CMHC is one of them.

The CMHC, with its academic missions, might be particularly vulnerable in the future given the costs of the academic programs in a time of budget stringency. State ownership and operation do not enable the CMHC to expand services in pursuit of new revenues. All collections for services at the CMHC return to the general fund of the state. In 2010, with implementation of parity of insurance coverage for psychiatric illnesses and implementation of measures from the PPAC Act going forward, private nonprofit agencies might well expand revenue-based services, grow, and become more equal in size to the CMHC. On the other hand, being state owned may protect the CMHC from change in other ways, to the extent that the Department of Mental Health and Addiction Services (DMHAS), the parent state agency, values the institutional programs and is prepared to protect and support them.

One view of the future profile of services for the CMHC follows. The CMHC, funded by general fund dollars, continues to provide safety net treatment services for a residual population of uninsured people. Also, it provides psychiatric consultation services to primary care and other mental health services with limited psychiatric professionals regarding complex, unstable patients with serious mental illness. The consultations integrate treatment and rehabilitation, mental health and substance-use services, and primary care. The CMHC manages and offers rehabilitative and recovery services, again supported by state general fund dollars. It offers categorically funded programs such as community-based forensic services (alternatives to incarceration, prison reentry programs), young adult services, and outreach to homeless mentally ill people. It manages a system and clinically supports residential programs, coordinating with the two general hospitals in the metropolitan area. It continues to manage the local service system for the purpose of integrating mental health and substance-use services, behavioral health and rehabilitation services, and behavioral health and primary care. As a function of background mainstreaming processes, it collaborates more closely with general hospitals and CHCs in New Haven.

Because it is a community mental health center that teaches new generations of mental health professionals in preparation for public psychiatry, the CMHC continues a commitment to ambulatory treatment services and, perhaps, to a small acute inpatient service, especially for the residual uninsured population. These services demonstrate evidence-based practice, building new models of care and innovation through clinical trials. The CMHC uses these services as a platform for education of psychiatric residents and other mental health professionals. Educational programs include training to take responsibility for the chronic medical conditions—such as hypertension, obesity, smoking addiction, metabolic syndrome, and diabetes—that plague people with serious mental illness. CMHC faculty staff members might consult for other agencies in the state system to help them address these tasks related to health care reform and transformation.

A previous volume on academic programs at the CMHC documents the vibrant educational and research missions of the institution, also considering future directions for them (Jacobs and Griffith, 2007). It is essential that these missions be integrated into the service mission of the institution (see chapter 3). The relationship among the missions raises an interesting question about the direction of the relationship. Here is a premise for the future of public psychiatry at the CMHC. In reciprocal relationships, public services and service development ought to significantly define the academic missions of research and education, just as much as discovery and education change and shape services. In short, an academic community mental health center cannot function as an ivory tower.

Indeed the institution of the CMHC, the reflection of a partnership between the State of Connecticut and Yale University, is part of two worlds, the DMHAS of Connecticut and the Yale Department of Psychiatry (YDP) of the Yale School of Medicine. The challenge to the institution is to make itself indispensable to both the DMHAS and the YDP in meeting future needs for innovation and change. A remarkable array of services positions the institution to contribute to innovation. In the past two decades, Law and Psychiatry, the Division of Substance Abuse, and Recovery and Community Health have already done so. Additional academic programs are poised to move the institution forward, including Latino services, Young Adult Services, Problem Gambling, and co-occurring disorders programs. The challenge ahead involves a

> The challenge ahead involves a process of continuous adaptation to new challenges.

process of continuous adaptation to new challenges such as the integration of primary care and early intervention in initial episodes of psychosis. It is difficult to know exactly where the field of public psychiatry will end up in 10 or 20 years. A full spectrum of salient academic programs insures that the major bases are covered. In the meantime, academic programs make substantial contributions to the resource base of public psychiatry. Examples are residential resources and medical interventions already under study, supported by grant funds. Also, in each of the academic areas identified above, faculty and staff at the CMHC offer policy expertise to support decision making at a state level in the DMHAS, the federal level at the SAMHSA and the NIMH.

There is a perpetual challenge to inspire and educate new generations of public psychiatrists and other mental health professionals. In this regard the institution, in collaboration with the DMHAS, continues to offer an advanced, postdoctoral fellowship in public psychiatry. In addition, the CMHC continues research education regarding chronic illness to provide a foundation for academic careers in the public arena. In participation with other academic centers, a challenge for the future is to move toward added qualifications in public psychiatry

A consequence of the forces of change discussed in this chapter may be to orient the institution back towards a specialized "institute" model, in collaboration with DMHAS, to preserve, develop, and improve services for people with serious mental illness and for other target populations. This idea is not to suggest the CMHC would become an ivory tower, as the institution would still have to maintain a full spectrum of productive clinical services. Also, the institution might shoulder responsibility to consult for other state owned institutions. An institute model would have to include a responsibility and an opportunity to preserve and demonstrate services, especially innovative interventions, for populations served by programs of the state mental health authority. If return to such a model for the CHMC occurs, the institution would have come full circle, as the original concept that in 1957 set in motion its development was that of an institute.

State ownership and operation has served the CMHC well over the decades. While there have been ups and downs, the State of Connecticut has underwritten an academic institution for public psychiatry throughout the modern era. Though not exactly what Dr. Redlich envisaged when he met with Governor Ribicoff in 1957, somehow the CMHC has survived and worked over the years. In a national perspective, the CMHC is now virtually unique. It might serve as a model for other states in a new era.

EVOLVING VISIONS OF THE CONNECTICUT MENTAL HEALTH CENTER

Several visions of the future have guided the development of public psychiatry at the CMHC over the years. Political and economic realities repeatedly intruded. At the outset, the prevailing vision was for the CMHC to be an academic institute of psychiatry. Along came the community mental health movement that dominated developments. Early in the history of the CMHC, in the circumstances of conflict between academic and service missions, the CMHC leadership implemented a compromise, creating urgent care and crisis intervention. The new clinical organization, designed to provide high volume services at the front door while preserving academic programs for treatment, prevailed for many years. Then, the community services and systems movement for people with serious and persistent mental illness intruded. Unfortunately, a crisis in leadership at the CMHC aggravated a lagging attention to this change in public psychiatry. In its aftermath, it was necessary to reestablish the integrity of the institution, reestablish the partnership of the State of Connecticut and Yale University, and rebuild the institution, in part by catching up with community support programs. Key academic programs helped lead the CMHC out of this troubled time, just as they supported the institution in good times. Back on its feet, the CMHC then had to meet the challenges of mainstreaming, managed care, privatization, and transformation. Then, along came health care reform of 2010. In this text, the four periods of modern public psychiatry and, perhaps, a new period opening up, have served as organizational concepts for understanding this evolution in vision. The institution has thrived over the long haul by monitoring policy and environmental change and adapting as nimbly as possible, while preserving its core identity.

At the present time, the CMHC is a vibrant academic community mental health center that since 1966 has fulfilled the original vision establishing the three-part mission of services, education, and research. It is an admirable institution that (with apologies to Pascal) sustains a passionate commitment to understanding the infinitely small through molecular research and the infinitely large through mental health services research and the evolution of services in response to the needs of the people it serves, while adapting to the evolving context of mental health knowledge and policy. By embodying the best in services (especially for people with serious mental illness), and by pointing to the future with education and research, the CMHC continues to contribute to public psychiatry. Moving into the future, the admonition and exhortation of Dr. Redlich, delivered after having defined the challenging multiple missions of the academic CMHC, still resonate for those who work there: "More is expected of the Connecticut Mental Health Center."

CONCLUSION

This book has traced the history and the development of services at the CMHC during its institutional life. The book places the story of the CMHC in the context of mental health policy and movements over the modern era. During the post–World War II period mental health advocates set in motion the modern era, which is characterized by deinstitutionalization. At that time, cyclical concern in American society about overcrowded, and sometimes deplorable, conditions of many state psychiatric hospitals peaked again. After the Community Mental Health Act of 1963, community mental health centers started up across the country as part of a long process of development of community-based mental health services.

The contemporary picture of public psychiatry is quite different and characterized by multiple variables that are shaping its future. Still, vestiges of institutionalization persist in the chronic care of many people with serious mental illness in nursing homes. Even some special rehabilitation programs in the community, which do not strive for full participation and membership in the community, have an institutional quality. Health care reform probably will change that, as it pursues goals that were first formulated during the periods of mainstreaming and transformation in modern public psychiatry. Mainstreaming can be seen as the ultimate expression of deinstitutionalization. Yet while following the public debate on health care reform during 2009-10, it was interesting how little special attention was given to exceptional programs for people with serious mental illness. Rather, the major factors affecting change in public psychiatry in the contemporary scene touch all of health care and integrate not only patient care but also the public psychiatric system even more tightly into the mainstream of general health care.

If the point of view in this book is true about the huge changes in store for public psychiatry under health care reform, it makes it all the more important to have psychiatrists and other mental health professionals who have special preparation, knowledge, and commitment, to serve people with serious mental illness and disabilities, who are recovering and living in the community. More important than ever as the field of public psychiatry moves forward under mainstream assumptions, is the role of mental health professionals as leaders of a multidisciplinary mental health team that develops comprehensive plans of care in the community. It is a challenging and exciting time to practice in the public arena at present. It is a time of great opportunity related to expanded access to psychiatric services for people with mental illness. It is also a time to pay attention to the unfolding changes and to advocate for the treatment and rehabilitative services needed by people with serious mental illness as part of the mainstream health and welfare benefits in American society.

Bibliography

American Hospital Association, Behavioral Health Task Force Report, 2007 (September), http://www.aha.org/aha/issues/Mental-Health-Services/taskforcereport.html

Astrachan BM, The pragmatics of health delivery, Connecticut Medicine, 37, 1774-79, 1974

Astrachan BM, Tischler GT, A systems approach to the management of psychiatric facilities, Administration in Mental Health, 8, 225-39, 1981

Boston Globe, January 20, 2006

Brown DB, Goldman CR, Thompson KS, Cutler DL, Training residents for community psychiatric practice: guidelines for curriculum development, Community Mental Health Journal, 29, 271-83, 1993

Buck JA, Medicaid, healthcare financing trends, and the future of state-based public mental health services, Psychiatric Services, 54, 969-73, 2003

Cohen CI, Feiner JS, Huffine C, Moffic HS, Thompson KS, The future of community psychiatry, Community Mental Health Journal, 39, 459-71, 2003

Community Mental Health Journal, Special Issue Commemorating the Anniversary of the Community Mental Health Centers Act of 1963, 39, 2003

Cutler D, Bevilacqua J, McFarland B, Four decades of community mental health: a symphony in four movements, Community Mental Health, 39(5), 381-98, 2003

Dailey WF, Kirk TA, Cole RA, DiLeo PJ, Public academic partnership at the Connecticut Mental Health Center, In 40 Years of Academic Public Psychiatry, Jacobs SC, Griffith EEH (eds), John Wiley and Sons, 2007

Davidson L, Living Outside Mental Illness: Qualitative Studies of Recovery in Schizophrenia, New York, New York University Press, 2003

Davidson L, Harding CM, Spaniol L, Recovery from Severe Mental Illnesses: Research Evidence and Implications for Practice, Volume 1, Boston, MA, Center for Psychiatric Rehabilitation of Boston University, 2005

Davidson L, Harding CM, Spaniol L, Recovery from Severe Mental Illnesses: Research Evidence and Implications for Practice, Volume 2, Boston, MA, Center for Psychiatric Rehabilitation of Boston University, 2006

Drake RE, Green AI, Muesser KT, Goldman HH, The history of community health treatment and rehabilitation for persons with severe mental illness, Community Mental Health Journal, 39, 427-40, 2003

Foley HA, Sharfstein SS, Madness and Government: Who Cares for the Mentally Ill, Washington, DC, American Psychiatric Press, 1983

Frank RG, Glied SA, Better But Not Well: Mental Health Policy in the United States Since 1950, Baltimore, the Johns Hopkins University Press, 2006

Frank RG, Goldman HH, Hogan M, Medicaid and mental health: be careful what you ask for, Health Affairs, 22, 201-13, 2003

Georgetown University Health Policy Institute, Center for Children and Families, Medicaid and state budgets: looking at the facts, April, 2008, http://ccf.georgetown.edu

Glied SA, Frank RG, Better but not well, recent trends in the well being of the mentally ill, Health Affairs, 28, 637-48, 2009

Goldman HH, The obligation of mental health services to the least well off, Psychiatric Services, 50, 659-64, 1999

Governor's Hospital System Strategic Task Force Report, State of Connecticut, January 8, 2008, http://www.ct.gov/ohca/lib/ohca/taskforce/hospitaltask-force/hospital_task_force_master_version_1-17-08.pdf

Grob GN, From Asylum to Community: Mental Health Policy in Modern America, Princeton, NJ, Princeton University Press, 1991

Grob GN, Goldman HH, The Dilemma of Federal Mental Health Policy: Radical Reform or Incremental Change, New Brunswick NJ, Rutgers University Press, 2007

Harding CM, Zubin J, Strauss JS, Chronicity in schizophrenia: fact, partial fact, or artifact, Hospital and Community Psychiatry, 38, 77-86, 1987

Insel TR, Fenton WS, Psychiatric epidemiology: it is not just about counting any more, Archives of General Psychiatry, 62, 590-92, 2005

Insel TR, Translating scientific opportunity into public health impact: a strategic plan for research on mental illness, Archives of General Psychiatry, 66, 128-39, 2009

Institute of Medicine, Crossing the Quality Chasm: A New Health System for the 21st Century, Washington, DC, National Academy Press, 2001

Jacobs SC, 50 Years of Social and Community Psychiatry, October 23, 1998, unpublished lecture manuscript

Jacobs SC, Griffith EEH, 40 Years of Academic Public Psychiatry, London, John Wiley and Sons, 2007

Kaiser Family Foundation, Health Reform Implementation Timeline, April 10, 2010a, http://www.kff.org/healthreform/8060.cfm

Kaiser Family Foundation, Focus on Health Care Reform, Explaining Health Care Reform: Questions About Medicaid's Role, April, 20, 2010b, http://www.kff.org, publication #7920-02

Kirk TA, State of Connecticut, Department of Mental Health and Addiction Services, Announcement, June 19, 2009

Levinson DJ, Klerman GL, The Clinician-Executive, Psychiatry, 30, 3-14, 1967

Lieberman JA, Stroup TS, McEvoy JP, et al, Clinical antipsychotic trials of intervention effectiveness (CATIE): effectiveness of antipsychotic drugs in patients with chronic schizophrenia, New England Journal of Medicine, 353, 1209-23, 2005

Manderschied RW, Atay JE, Hernandez-Cartegena M, et al, Highlights of Organized Mental Health Services in 1998 in Major National and State Trends, Manderschied RW, Henderson MJ (eds), US Health and Human Services, Center for Mental Health Services, Rockville, SAMHSA, CMHS, 2000 (February) http://www.mentalhealth.org/publications/allpubs/ SMA01-3537/chapter4asp

Mark TL, Levit KR, Coffey RM, et al, National Expenditures for Mental Health Services and Substance Abuse Treatment, 1993-2003, USDHHS, SAMHSA, DHHS Publication No. SMA07-4227, 2007

Murray JL, Lopez, AD (eds), Global Burden of Disease, Cambridge, MA, Harvard University Press, 1996

National Association of State Mental Health Program Directors (NASMHPD) Medical Directors Council, Parkes J, Svendsen D, Singer P, Foti ME (eds), Morbidity and mortality in people with serious mental illness, http://www.nasmhpd.org, October, 2006

National Council for Community Behavioral Health (NCCBH), Summary of the Major Provisions of the PPAC Act, April 7, 2010a, http://www.thenationalcouncil.org

National Council for Community Behavioral Health, Health Care Reform: Getting Down to Business, Letter from Linda, April 13, 2010b, http://www.thenationalcouncil.org

Open Minds, Online News, Medicaid to become 35% of state budgets by 2030, July 2, 2010

Power AK, A public health model of mental health for the 21st century, Psychiatric Services, 60, 580-84, 2009

President's New Freedom Commission on Mental Health, 2003, http://www.mentalhealthcommission.gov/reports/reports.htm

Ranz JM, Deakins SM, Lemelle SM, Rosenheck SD, Kellerman SL, Core elements of a public psychiatry fellowship, Psychiatric Services, 718-20, 2008

Ranz JM, Demographic analysis of members of the American Association of Community Psychiatrists, Community Mental Health Journal, 40, 479-86, 2004

Ranz JM, Vergare MJ, Wilk E, et al, The tipping point from private practice to publicly funded settings for early- and mid-career psychiatrists, Psychiatric Services, 57, 1640-43, 2006

Raylesberg DD, Action for Mental Health: Final Report of he Joint Commission on Mental Illness and Health 1961, New York, Basic Books, 1961

Redlich FC, Preface, In The University and Community Mental Health, New Haven, Yale University Press, 1966

Rosenberg L, Testimony to Congress, 2009, http://www.thenationalcouncil.org/cs/press_releases/mental_health_and_addictions_safety_net_in_crisis

Ryan W, Blaming the Victim. Random House, New York, 1971

Sowers WE, Thompson KS, (eds), Keystones for Collaboration and Leadership: Issues and Recommendations for the Transformation of Community Psychiatry, American Association of Community Psychiatrists, 2007, http://www.communitypsychiatry.org (Transformation report)

Sledge WH, Tebes J, Rakfeldt J, Davidson L, Lyons L, Druss B, Day hospital/ crisis respite care versus inpatient care, part I: clinical outcomes, American Journal of Psychiatry, 153, 1065-73, 1996a

Sledge WH, Tebes J, Wolff N, Helminiak TW, Day hospital/crisis respite care versus inpatient care, part II: service utilization and costs, American Journal of Psychiatry, 153, 1074-83, 1996b

Stein LI, Test MA, Alternative to mental hospital treatment: I. conceptual model, treatment program, and clinical evaluation. Archives of General Psychiatry, 37, 392-97, 1980

Steinhauer J, To cut costs states relax prison policies, New York Times, March 25, 2009

Strauss JS, Hafez H, Lieberman RP, et al, The course of psychiatric disorder, III: longitudinal principles, American Journal of Psychiatry, 142, 289-96, 1985

Tischler GL, Henisz J, Myers J, Catchmenting and the use of mental health services, Archives of General Psychiatry, 27, 89-92, 1972a

Tischler GL, Henisz J, Myers J, et al, The impact of catchmenting, Administration in Mental Health, 1, 22-29, 1972b

Tischler GL, Henisz J, Myers J, et al, The utilization of mental health services, III: mediators of service allocation, Archives of General Psychiatry, 32, 416-28, 1975

Turner JC, Tenhoor WJ, The NIMH community support program: pilot approach to a needed social reform, Schizophrenia Bulletin, 4, 310-49, 1978

U.S. Department of Health and Human Services, Towards a National Plan for the Chronically Mentally Ill, Rockville, MD, USDHHS, 1980

U.S. Department of Health and Human Services, Public Health Service, Mental Health: A Report of the Surgeon General, Rockville, MD, USDHHS, SAMHSA, CMS, NIH, NIMH, 1999a

U.S. Department of Health and Human and Human Services, The Surgeon General's Call to Action to Prevent Suicide, 1999b, http://www.surgeongeneral.gov/library/calltoaction/calltoaction.htm

U.S. Department of Health and Human and Human Services, Public Health Service, Mental Health: Culture, Race, and Ethnicity, A Supplement to Mental Health: A Report of the Surgeon General, 2001, http://www.surgeongeneral.gov/library/mentalhealth/cre/

Wexler B, Davidson L, Styron T, Strauss J, Severe and persistent mental illness, Chapter 1, In 40 Years of Pubic Psychiatry Jacobs SC, Griffith EEH (eds), London, Wiley and Sons, 2007

Wyatt v. Stickney, 325 F. Supp. 781 (Ala. 1971), 334 F. Supp. 1341 (Ala. 1971), 344 F. Supp. 373 (Ala. 1972)

Yedida MJ, Gillespie CC, Bernstein CA, A survey of psychiatric residency directors on current priorities and preparation for public sector care, Psychiatric Services, 57, 238-43, 2006

Zeichner AM, The origins of the Connecticut Mental Health Center, unpublished manuscript, June 16, 1970

Index